MEDICINE'S NEW TECHNOLOGY:
A Career Guide

MEDICINE'S NEW

Janet Zhun Nassif

TECHNOLOGY:

A Career Guide

ARCO PUBLISHING, INC.
NEW YORK

For Fred
Who makes it all happen

Published by Arco Publishing, Inc.
219 Park Avenue South, New York, N.Y. 10003

Library of Congress Cataloging in Publication Data
Nassif, Janet Zhun.
  Medicine's new technology.

  1. Biomedical technicians—Vocational guidance.
2. Biomedical engineering—Vocational guidance.
I. Title.
R856.25.N37   610   78–11386

ISBN 0–668–04443–8 (Library Edition)

Printed in the United States of America

Contents

Acknowledgments

This book is about health professionals and could not have been written without their assistance. Thanks to Mimi Berman RDMS, Assistant Professor, Radiological Sciences and Technology Program, College of Health Related Professions, Downstate Medical Center; Louise Botto RN, Director, School of Operating Room Technology, Columbia Presbyterian Medical Center; James Giebfried PT, New York University Medical Center; Robert Guthrie, Chief Technologist, Cardiac Laboratory, New York University Medical Center; Francine Hekelman RN, Director, Education Committee, American Association of Nephrology Nurses and Technicians; Ruth Jackson RCT, President, American Cardiology Technologists Association; Mark I. Muilenburg CNMT, Past President, Society of Nuclear Medicine; Horatio Pineda MD, Pulmonary Laboratory, New York University Medical Center; James Stephens CORT, Director of Education, Association of Operating Room Technicians; and to the other professionals whose names appear elsewhere in this book.

Also to John Acuff, National Society for Cardiopulmonary Technology; Antoinette Alesi, Downstate Medical Center; Anne Allen, Ohio State University; Patricia Dedman, American Medical Association; Cecile French, OR Tech; Irving Goldberg, Jerry Gordon, National Institutes of Health; Timothy Keane, Medical Systems Division, General Electric Co.; Diane Lynch, American Cancer Society; Arlene Soodak, National Institutes of Health; James Warren, National Kidney Foundation; Myron Youdin, Institute of Rehabilitation Medicine, New York University Medical Center.

Special thanks to Marcia Lewicki for her enthusiasm, professionalism, and patience in typing this manuscript, and to my husband, Fred Nassif, for his constant help, encouragement, and support throughout this project, without whom this book would not have been written.

Foreword

Few people think of health as an industry, yet it is one of the largest and fastest-growing industries in the United States. More than 4,000,000 men and women work in health care in such settings as hospitals, nursing homes, clinics, neighborhood health centers, health maintenance organizations, group practices, voluntary health agencies, and other health-related institutions and organizations. No other industry offers career opportunities that are so diversified, and many of the most meaningful and rewarding jobs are found in the area of health technology.

Ten years ago no one ever heard of a respiratory therapist or diagnostic medical sonographer. By the mid-70's, both of these occupations were firmly established. They emerged because of developments in technology, consumer demands, and changes in the health care delivery system—job market influences inherent in the health care field.

Many people think that all jobs in technological areas require aptitude in mathematics and science. Some do and some don't. The only way to determine whether a job in technology is for you is to learn as much as possible about the requirements and qualifications for different occupations. What does a nuclear medicine technologist do? What kinds of skills and aptitudes are required for the biomedical engineer? How long will it take to become a radiographer? Is a dialysis technician licensed or certified? Answers to these and other questions are presented in this book.

After reading about the different technological jobs, follow up on the ones that interest you most by talking to persons actually employed as technicians or technologists. If possible, spend a few hours or days watching the person work. This is the best way to get a real feeling for the job. After narrowing your career choice to one or two possibilities, find out about the availability of educational programs in the area and look into the potential job market. Armed with the facts, you will be in a better position to make a satisfying career selection. So if a career in health technology appeals to you, read on.

Barbara I. Bloom
Director
Division of Career Information
American Hospital Association

MEDICINE'S NEW TECHNOLOGY:

A Career Guide

CHAPTER I

Your Future in
Medicine's New Technology

Within seconds, a slice of the brain can be produced by combining the magic of X-rays and the marvels of the computer. A special machine can substitute for your heart, lungs, or kidneys. Sonar, once used to probe the deep for enemy submarines during wartime, is now being used to hunt enemies lurking within the mysterious depths of our own bodies.

Medical marvels? Yes. Unusual? No. These exciting technological developments are common occurrences in medicine today. Since the discovery of X-rays, medicine has literally "taken off." And while outer space exploration may steal the headlines, the exploration of inner space, within our own bodies, offers one of the greatest adventures in the world of science and technology in the 1980's.

How you decide to join the great adventure is up to you. Though physicians traditionally have been in the foreground of this frontier, in today's medical world there are many other important health professionals who make a vital contribution behind the scenes.

Who are they? And what do they do? You will soon find out. They are: Profusionists, Operating Room Technicians, Nuclear Medicine Technologists, Diagnostic Medical Sonographers, Respiratory Therapists, and other health professionals. All are specialists who, in one way or another, make a vital contribution to health. They use their minds, their hands, their hearts, and medicine's new technology to assist in diagnosing or treating disease, sustaining or improving human life, or unravelling its mysteries.

Each chapter will introduce you to a different specialist. You will explore in depth the role these health professionals play in medicine today, observe them in action, and learn how you can join their special ranks.

Some of these professions take but months to earn, others several years; but most careers in medicine's new technology can be yours within just two years' time.

The word "technology" may give you the impression that these careers are complex and unattainable. But don't let a word scare you. Technology means nothing more than the "application of science," and in this book, science is applied to helping people in trouble get better. You don't have to be a scientific genius to do this. There are opportunities for persons with different levels of interest and ability. But no matter which career you select, you must be ready to put time, work, and effort into it; dedication is what medicine is all about. Judging from the remarks of the health professionals you will meet here, this dedication pays off.

So if you think you might like to put your talents to work in the health field, turn the page and discover if your future lies in medicine's new technology.

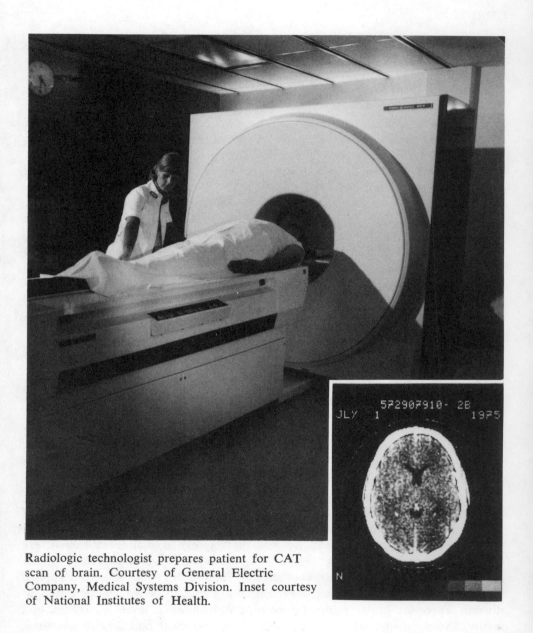

Radiologic technologist prepares patient for CAT scan of brain. Courtesy of General Electric Company, Medical Systems Division. Inset courtesy of National Institutes of Health.

CHAPTER II

X-Rays: The Birth of New Technology

It happened accidentally, less than 100 years ago in a small town on the other side of the world. A German scientist, Wilhelm Roentgen, had been working alone in a tiny laboratory for several weeks, when one winter night he made a startling discovery in the dark.

He had pitched his lab into total darkness in a test to find out whether a cardboard box he had constructed and placed over a vacuum tube would block all light produced by an electric current passing through the tube.

He turned on the current and watched. No light was visible from the tube, but something did catch his eye. Hovering mysteriously a few feet from the tube was a strange green cloud. He looked quickly around the room for the source of this phenomenon. Seeing none, he switched off the current. The green haze disappeared. Curious, he turned on the current again and the green cloud reappeared. Moving closer to the light he saw that this unusual effect was being created by the glistening of some barium crystals which had been left on the desk.

But what was causing the crystals to phosphorize? Roentgen knew of no energy source that could explain what was happening. This must be something new, something unknown and unnamed. It was then that he decided to call these strange rays X-rays, after the mathematical symbol "X," which stands for the unknown.

In the days that followed, Roentgen repeated his "accident" again, this time substituting a crystal screen for the barium crystals. He began to learn more about his mysterious X-rays. They could penetrate most material—heavy cloth, wood, and metals, except for platinum and lead. But when he passed his hand in front of the X-ray producing tube he received another surprise. Not only did the rays pass through his hand, but his hand was clearly silhouetted on the crystal screen. And it was not the mere outline of the hand; the inside detail of the bones and joints was clearly visible. Later he substituted a special photographic plate for the crystal screen and found he could actually produce an X-ray photograph.

Roentgen couldn't have known then, in 1895, that he had done more than just discover a strange new energy source. He had started a medical revolution. At

3

last a discovery had been made which, in the years to come, would move medicine from the realm of educated guesswork into the world of science and technology.

Today over two hundred million X-rays are performed annually, making X-ray examination a basic tool of health care.

WHO USES X-RAYS?

In the medical world the science of X-rays is called radiology. Many health practitioners—physicians, dentists, podiatrists, chiropractors, veterinarians—use X-rays to diagnose injury or illness. The jobs of the radiation therapy technologist and radiologic technologist are also intimately involved with X-ray use. You'll meet the radiation therapy technologist in the next chapter.

The radiologic technologist, formerly called an X-ray technician, uses X-rays to create radiographs, which are X-ray images of the human body. Physicians who specialize in interpreting X-ray and related imaging techniques are radiologists.

Unlike taking a regular photograph, performing an X-ray examination requires special skill and training. The radiologic technologist's job, as you will see, is much more than just picture-taking.

THE RADIOLOGIC TECHNOLOGIST AND THE PATIENT

Who receives X-ray examinations? Practically everybody. In fact, it's a rare adult today who has never had an X-ray examination. Radiologic technologists work with patients of all kinds, sick and healthy, old and young.

Some patients may have broken bones or other internal problems caused by accidents or injuries; others may have suspected ulcers, tumors, or growths. Still other patients who do not have any obvious problems undergo a routine X-ray exam as part of a comprehensive physical examination.

In many instances X-rays are used to evaluate special situations. For example, prior to surgery, X-rays can help locate a foreign object which has entered the body, whether it be a bullet in an adult or a toy which a child has accidentally swallowed.

Radiologic technology can be used to probe and photograph almost any internal organ or part of the human body, which is why it is considered a basic diagnostic tool in health care.

But whatever the reason for the X-ray, the radiologic technologist's basic responsibility remains the same—to produce a radiograph of the highest diagnostic quality while exposing the patient to the smallest radiation risk and causing the least discomfort.

To appreciate the complexities of the radiologic technologist's job, some basic knowledge of X-rays and how radiographs are produced is helpful.

THE ABC'S OF X-RAYS

Despite the tremendous advances in radiologic technology, most modern equipment produces X-rays in essentially the same manner as Roentgen's first crude X-ray machine. X-rays are generated when electrons, produced and moving at great speed inside a vacuum tube, are suddenly stopped by an object, usually a tungsten filament, inside the tube. Upon impact some energy is converted to heat, some into X-rays.

X-rays move at the speed of light and are similar to other energy forms, such as light waves or radio waves. X-rays, however, have a much higher energy level, and therefore can penetrate most objects. The higher the electric power, or voltage, producing the electrons, the higher the energy level and penetration of the resulting X-rays.

As Roentgen learned, X-rays, like light waves, can expose photographic film; but an X-ray picture is different. It is a negative image, actually a photographic record of the different tissue densities of the body. As the X-rays pass through the patient, some rays are absorbed. Just how much depends on the density of the body tissues. The thicker the tissues, the greater their density and ray absorption. Consequently, fewer rays reach and expose the photographic film, leaving a light area.

Without differing tissue densities, no image can be produced. For example, if a hand is X-rayed, the bones—which are much denser than surrounding tissues—will readily absorb X-rays and appear on the film as distinct white shapes. The individual muscles, nerves, and tendons of the hand, however, cannot be seen, since they, like all body tissues, have the same approximate densities. X-rays which pass through them will be absorbed equally. Without *contrasting* density they cannot be individually seen.

How then can an organ be radiographed? By artificially creating different densities in the organ and surrounding tissues.

Perhaps you have heard of a barium cocktail. This is a heavy but harmless mixture of barium salts. When swallowed by the patient, the barium creates this contrasting density in the stomach. Thus, when X-rayed, the stomach can be seen. Barium is just one of the methods used to produce contrast.

Air is a natural contrast medium. In a chest X-ray, for example, you will be asked to take a deep breath. The air entering the lungs creates stronger contrast with the surrounding tissues and produces a clearer radiograph. Air, as well as other gasses, such as oxygen, helium, and carbon dioxide, are used in other X-ray procedures. In pneumoencephalography, some spinal fluid is removed and replaced with air or gas so radiographs of the skull can be taken.

Special dyes are also used to produce tissue contrast. In performing an intravenous pyelogram, or IVP for short, the kidneys, bladder, and urethers can be seen on X-ray film after an iodine compound is injected into the veins. Depending on how much dye is absorbed (as observed on the X-ray film), it is possible to tell if obstructions or other abnormalities in these areas are present.

With an understanding of these X-ray basics, let's look at what the radiologic technologist must consider in order to produce that quality radiograph.

TAKING AN X-RAY

If you have ever had a medical X-ray taken, the radiologic technologist's job may have seemed deceptively simple. Just position the patient, film, and X-ray equipment. Then adjust a few dials and finally push a button.

What wasn't apparent was the many varied factors involved in producing a quality radiograph.

The first and most important element is proper density. If too much or too little density is present, the radiograph, like a photograph, will appear either under- or over-exposed.

Next, good contrast is needed. The differences between tissue densities must be clearly visible. Still other variables are involved; even with proper density and good contrast, the image will be useless if it is not distinct and without distortion.

Unless the technologist can balance all these elements, the resulting radiograph will be of little or no diagnostic value to the radiologist. Achieving this balance requires skill, judgment, and the juggling of many technical factors.

The technologist must first look at the particular radiograph that is requested and then quickly size up the patient. Depending on the type of the exam which has been ordered, the individual patient's size can be very important. Is the patient tall and thin or short and stocky? Are the muscles well developed? Remember, different tissues thicknesses will affect the radiograph. Disease can affect body tissues, and consequently the X-ray film. Therefore, for some X-ray exams the patient's overall medical condition must be assessed. A fluid-filled lung, for example, X-rays differently from a normal lung.

Can the patient cooperate with the exam or is he or she likely to move suddenly, without warning, and blur the image?

Safety also must be considered. The radiation risk to the patient must be minimized while still achieving a good radiograph.

After weighing all these factors, the examination still cannot begin. The technologist must first adjust the distance between the X-ray beam and the patient, properly align the patient, and then determine the proper kilovoltage (kvp) and milliamperes (ma) and the number of seconds the patient will be exposed to the X-ray beam.

Although equipment charts can guide the technologist in determining the proper control settings, no chart can possibly reflect each situation that will be encountered with each new patient. Adapting the chart to each circumstance depends on the technologist's experience, skill, and radiographic art.

You have already seen some of the purely technical factors which are necessary to produce a good diagnostic film. But the human factors in this profession are equally important.

THE HUMAN ELEMENT

Throughout the X-ray exam, the radiologic technologist works closely with the patient. Good communication is where the patient contact begins. The patient must understand what kind of radiographic exam is needed, any preparation that is necessary, what will happen during the exam, and how he or she will be expected to cooperate.

Most patients, if they understand what is happening, will cooperate—and this cooperation can make a big difference in the film which is produced. The patient who understands that even slight movement, as little as one quarter millimeter, can cause X-ray distortion may help the technologist avoid retakes.

To guard against movement, sandbags or other devices are often used to immobilize the body part which will be X-rayed. If the patient can't cooperate, as in the case of an unconscious, confused, or senile patient, or in the case of a small child, the technologist must use special techniques to compensate for probable movement of the patient.

Although X-rays are totally painless and cannot be felt, many of the X-ray procedures can be unpleasant for the patient. Some patients may simply be in pain, whether it be from broken bones, disease, or internal injuries. Any body movement or touching may cause them discomfort. The use of contrast media may cause a patient some physical distress. Before a contrast medium can be introduced into the patient, advance preparation is usually necessary. The patient may be required the forgo food and drink for several hours. The patient may also be requested to take special cathartic substances to completely clean out the body. (This helps insure that the contrast medium, when introduced, will more clearly outline all the internal structures.) After preparation, the patient may feel weak or nauseous. The technologist must be sensitive to the patient's needs and, where possible, try to minimize patient discomfort.

When contrast media is used in a radiologic examination, the technologist must exercise extra care and precautions. Certain contrast dyes or other substances used in some X-ray procedures may cause an allergic reaction in a small percentage of patients. The reaction may range from a mild itching or stinging of the skin to a serious one during which the patient's breathing may stop and death could occur. Because there is no way of predicting how a patient will react, the technologist must always be alert to any changes in the patient's condition, even those which the patient may disregard as unimportant.

But the human element of the job doesn't end with the patient. Radiologic technologists work with other health professionals too, primarily doctors and nurses.

Most physician contact is with the supervising radiologist of the X-ray department. Many special X-ray procedures require that the radiologic technologist and radiologist work together as a team. Fluoroscopy is one such area where teamwork is required.

Fluoroscopy differs from the conventional X-ray exam in that the patient is positioned against a special screen instead of X-ray film. With the use of contrast media, the physician can view the internal organs in action on the fluorescent screen.

Bedside radiography brings the technologist and nurse together. When the patient is too ill to travel to the X-ray department or too encumbered with traction devices or other medical paraphernalia, the technologist goes to the patient. Because the nurse in charge is responsible for everything that happens on the patient floor, he or she must be notified when an X-ray exam has been ordered and is going to take place. Through the nurse, the technologist can gain much valuable information about any aspect of the patient's condition which could affect the exam. Bedside examinations present a special challenge for the radiologic technologist because normal radiographic procedures must usually be modified to meet the unique demands of the patient's situation.

Whether it be at the patient's bedside, in the hospital X-ray department, or in the emergency or operating room, the radiologic technologist's duties do not end with the X-ray exam itself. Let's look beyond the exam to the technologist's other responsibilities.

ADDITIONAL DUTIES

Like any other film, the X-ray must be developed, either manually or by automatic processing. Though the majority of the work is done automatically, the technologist must be thoroughly knowledgeable about film processing and be prepared to do this manually if the proper equipment is not available. Once developed, the film will have to be reviewed for proper imaging. Is the image clear and distinct? Is proper contrast present? Does the radiograph provide the necessary diagnostic information? Though the radiologist is not responsible for interpreting the film itself, technologists must decide whether or not the film is good enough to be of value to the radiologist. If the technologist deems the quality poor, a retake will be necessary. But before that can be done, the technologist must decide where the fault lies. Was it the technique? Should the controls be adjusted? Or is the equipment malfunctioning?

Making this determination requires knowledge of equipment basics. The technologists must be able to spot whether poor radiographic quality is due to machine malfunction or improper techniques. Though the equipment manufacturer is responsible for equipment maintenance, minor equipment problems cannot wait for their biomedical equipment technicians. Technologists must be able to make minor on-the-spot repairs so as not to seriously delay department operations.

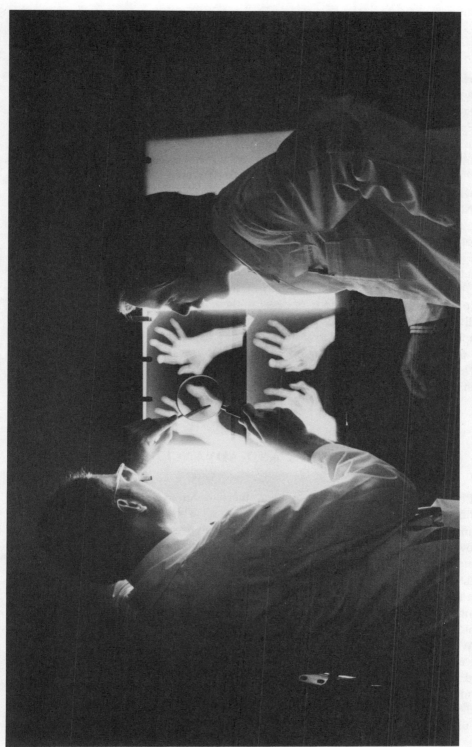

Physicians depend on X-rays for diagnosis. Here the physician and radiologic technologist examine X-rays of patients' hands with rheumatoid arthritis. Courtesy of National Institutes of Health.

If the film is of good quality, it becomes a permanent and valued part of the patient's record. Accurate record keeping in X-ray is extremely important. A mismarked film could cause an error in diagnosis. Accuracy is important for another reason: the X-ray film, like other parts of the patient's record, is frequently used as evidence in malpractice or other injury suits.

Each radiograph must be clearly labeled with basic information identifying the patient and information that outlines the pertinent details of the exam. This would include data on the various equipment control settings, the patient's position during the exam, and an exact anatomical statement identifying the body part which has been radiographed.

All films must be carefully handled and stored to preserve film quality and prevent deterioration. An X-ray film may be used for many years, for comparison or other reasons.

Finally, the technologist has general administrative duties. No department can function without organizing supplies and scheduling—both patients and department employees. Depending on the position of the technologist within the department, he or she must assume more or less of these administrative responsibilities. In addition, senior technologists usually have general teaching duties within the hospital. For example, they may instruct X-ray department personnel in techniques for personal and patient radiation safety.

Now that you have seen the basic responsibilities of this profession, let's look briefly at special areas in this changing technological field.

SPECIAL PROCEDURES AND ADVANCED TECHNOLOGY

Beyond basic radiologic technology, there is an exciting area referred to by radiologic professionals as "Special Procedures." This encompasses a broad spectrum of radiologic procedures requiring technologists who possess superior skills in overall radiographic techniques, whether it be patient positioning, making special equipment adjustments, or adapting the examination for particularly difficult patients. A special procedure technologist must be capable not only of working as a team member closely allied with the radiologist and carrying out highly complex examinations, but also of wc.king independently when necessary. Pneumoencephalography, previously mentioned, is an example of a special procedure.

Within the category of special procedures lie some of the most interesting and innovative uses of technology in medicine today. The "CAT" scanner—computerized axial tomography, CAT for short—introduced as recently as 1972 is a primary example. In just a short time the CAT has literally revolutionized diagnosis and patient monitoring in neurology and neurosurgery. In involves rapid scanning of the head by a narrow X-ray beam, coupled with a computer. The computer then translates the differences in tissue density detected along the beam path into numerical or pictorial displays. This technique is 100 times more sensitive than conventional X-ray procedures. It also produces better imaging of the various brain structures, eliminating the need for some traditional X-ray methods which are more dangerous for the patient and cause a great deal of patient discomfort. With the CAT, the entire brain can be scanned in less than five minutes. The computer generates oscilloscope-like images, similar to TV pictures, which reproduce cross sections of brain tissue structure as if the brain itself had been laid open at each successive level for viewing. Hence, the word "axial," meaning cross section, and "tomograph," meaning slice. Literally, the CAT produces a cross-sectional slice of the human body. But the CAT is not limited to brain scanning; it can produce slices of other parts of the human body as well.

Although the CAT is the most sophisticated radiologic equipment used today, it exposes the patient to less radiation than conventional X-rays.

But the CAT scanner is just one example of advancing radiologic technology.

The Xerox Corporation, the original manufacturer of office duplicating machines which revolutionized secretarial work, is now moving into biomedical technology as well. Their newly developed technique, Xeroradiography, uses special X-ray equipment and radiographic plates rather than traditional X-ray film. This technique gives much better pictures of certain kinds of body tissues, such as breast tissue, than regular X-ray film. This technique may eventually replace traditional mammography, which is X-ray examination of the breast. Though mammography has been taught for many years as a basic X-ray technique, with increasing emphasis on early detection of breast cancer, mammography in many hospitals today constitutes a "special" procedure.

Thermography is another area which is proving valuable in early detection of breast cancers. Thermography differs from mammography in that a thermograph is not an X-ray at all, but an image of the body produced by picking up and recording the heat given off by body tissues. Thermography is useful in detecting breast cancer because cancerous tissues generally emit higher heat energy than noncancerous areas. By identifying "hot" spots, as seen on the thermogram, the physician can spot a possible cancer. Though the technique is not absolutely foolproof, thermography can be an extremely useful diagnostic tool when used in conjunction with other traditional methods of diagnosis, such as physical examination.

Diagnostic medical sonography is another example of nonradioactive imaging in growing use today. Because sonography is an "imaging" technique, creating diagnostic pictures by sound waves rather than radiation, many working in the field today have come from the related science of radiologic technology. (See Chapter V, "Seeing With Sound.")

The effects of these new special procedures and of advanced technology on the radiologic field are difficult to predict. One fact is certain: These techniques are here to stay and their use is increasing rapidly. Many may eventually replace conventional X-ray methods.

AN AVERAGE DAY

It's 7:30 A.M. The outside world is still quiet, but inside your world, the hospital world, the radiologic technology department is already bustling with activity. You have already reviewed the day's full work schedule. Several of the patients on your schedule today are "outpatients," patients seen in the department who are not hospitalized. You silently hope your outpatients will be on time today so the day will run smoothly.

Several GI series' (X-ray studies of the gastrointestinal tract) are scheduled for the morning, so you mix a large batch of barium "cocktails." Your first examination, however, is a simple chest X-ray which is routinely required for all patients admitted to your hospital. The patient, Mr. Redell, hasn't been assigned to his room yet, so he is still in "civilian" attire. A department aide should have already instructed the patient to remove all metal objects from the chest area, but you double-check anyway. Anything that goes wrong with the examination will be your responsibility. Sure enough, he has forgotten some loose change in his pocket.

He questions the need for the examination. After all, he says, what does a chest X-ray have to do with the leg operation for which he is being admitted? You smile. You have answered this question many times before to different patients. You patiently explain that unexpected respiratory ailments can develop in any patient, but especially those undergoing operations. This X-ray can provide valuable diagnostic information later if any such problems arise.

All the time you have been talking to Mr. Redell you have been assessing his body type. He is stocky, with heavy muscles and a large barrel chest. You will have to adjust the standard X-ray setting in order to get the best X-ray for this patient. You carefully calculate the changes necessary, reset the controls, and then position the patient. You instruct him on breathing for the exam and caution him not to move. You quickly move behind the glassed-in control area. Seconds later the exam is completed. You ask him to wait outside until the film is developed and you are sure that it is satisfactory.

The X-ray is good; Mr. Redell leaves.

You start setting up your next examination, a radiologic examination of the upper and lower GI tract. The patient, Mrs. Crosby, has anemia. Her physician has ordered these examinations to determine if an ulcer or other intestinal problem may be the cause.

During the upper GI, Mrs. Crosby will have to drink a barium cocktail. You take the pitcher that you mixed earlier and carefully measure the right amount into a tall glass. You then ask the department clerk to pull any previous GI X-rays which may be on file for this patient. If any are available, you know the radiologist will want to review the previous studies for comparison. You then move the fluoroscopy unit into place and adjust the control panel. Using a push button, you change the massive examination table from its usual horizontal position into an upright one for the first part of the examination. Your preparation is almost complete. You don a heavy lead apron which will protect you from excess radiation and dim the lights. Now you are ready for your patient.

A nurse's aide wheels Mrs. Crosby into the examination room. You help her out of the wheelchair. Though you have performed this examination hundreds of times before, you realize that this exam may be Mrs. Crosby's first, so you take care to explain the procedure in detail. You tell her exactly what will happen and how she can assist you and the radiologist during the examination. Why is it so dark in here? she asks. You explain that like any motion picture, the fluoroscopic image is easier to see if it is viewed in a darkened room. While you are positioning her behind a fluoroscopic unit, Dr. Marshall, the radiologist, enters. He also puts on a heavy lead apron and lead gloves to protect his hands from X-rays while he is positioning the patient during the actual course of the examination.

The examination begins. You turn the unit on and hand the barium cocktail to Mrs. Crosby. Dr. Marshall instructs her to drink a small amount while he follows its progress on the screen as it travels from her esophagus to the stomach. A fluoroscopic image is the reverse of an X-ray; on the screen her stomach appears as a dark shape, rather than a light image as it would in an X-ray. Dr. Marshall continues to observe what is happening on the screen. He then asks you to take a series of X-rays and leaves to see his next patient.

You remove the fluoroscopy equipment and reposition your patient. You then quickly prepare for the radiologic examination. Now you use a caliper, a two-legged adjustable instrument similar to a protractor, to obtain an accurate measurement of her midsection. Based on the measurement, you select your control settings. To protect her from unnecessary radiation you take several steps: first, you select the proper film size, one which will expose just the necessary parts of the abdomen and no more; next, you add a special film grid and diaphragm and adjust the X-ray beam size. This filters out unnecessary radiation and prevents scattering of X-rays to other parts of the body. Because you are working with new equipment, a special cone which dramatically reduces excess radiation does not have to be added. It is a standard operating feature on your equipment. You are almost ready to begin. You add one more final protection measure—a lead shield that will help protect her reproductive organs from irradiation during the examination.

You move behind the glassed-in area and take the X-ray. You repeat the procedure several times, each time going back to your patient, reloading the film cassette, repositioning her, and finally taking the X-ray. When the radiographic study is complete, you tell Mrs. Crosby she can relax. Now she may take whatever position she wants until the film is developed and you are satisfied with its quality. Film processing in your department, as in most large hospitals today, is done automatically. A short time later they are ready. You quickly clip them to a lighted screen and check them carefully. The diagnostic quality is good. No retakes will be necessary.

You return to your patient and prepare her for the lower GI examination. You explain the procedure to Mrs. Crosby as you mix the barium preparation which will be given to her via an enema. You assemble the tubing and the enema bag, applying a lubricant to the tip of the tube. You reassure her that the procedure will not hurt, but that she will experience an unusual sense of fullness in her rectum. Dr. Marshall returns. You reposition the fluoroscopy equipment, drape the patient, and begin the procedure. During this part of the fluoroscopy exam you will be giving the barium enema and carefully controlling the flow of barium into the lower GI tract, while the radiologist observes its process on the screen. The exam goes uneventfully. Mrs. Crosby complains of tremendous pressure. You reassure her that the examination is almost over. Dr. Marshall leaves, again instructing you to expose a few radiographs. You know your patient is in discomfort and you move as quickly as possible to set up the radiologic exam. Within brief minutes you have taken the films. Mrs. Crosby uses the bathroom while you develop the film. These too are good. Mrs. Crosby can now return to her room while you finish your recordkeeping.

As you are just completing your last notation, the chief technologist enters and asks you to report immediately with a portable X-ray unit to the emergency room. A bus full of passengers has skidded off the road and overturned, and the injured are being brought in. You are pleased to have been chosen for this special duty. Generally emergency room work is reserved for the most skilled technologists because in emergency circumstances there is little time for retakes. Positioning patients who are critically injured also presents a challenge. Technologists must be creative in adapting standard positions to examine these patients.

The scene that greets you at the emergency room would appear chaotic to a nonprofessional. Nurses, doctors, and orderlies are moving quickly in all directions. Patients are being brought in on stretchers and a triage nurse meets them at the door, to determine the seriousness of their injuries. Hospitals do not use a first-come first-served basis for emergency medical care. In a triage ("three") system the most critically ill patients, whose lives are in immediate danger, are seen first. Next come patients who may be very ill or injured but are in "stable" condition. Those who need only routine or minor medical assistance are seen last.

An orderly spots you and says a back room will double as an X-ray room. Within a few seconds you are setting up for your first patient. An aide brings in a stretcher carrying a teenage girl. "Probably head trauma, suspected hip and pelvis fractures," he barks. You quickly check the patient's identification tag. Nancy Ellsworth. Though she is only semiconscious and moaning with pain, you call her by her first name. Even patients who are not fully aware of their surroundings can be reassured by this simple gesture. You will do the skull series first, since this is the most critical of her suspected injuries. You position her gently, using several sandbags to keep her head immobilized. You adjust the control setting so a shorter, more intensive X-ray will be used. This will help compensate for any involuntary movement by the patient and help prevent blurring. Once the skull series is finished, you place the film cassette in the basket, and an aide quickly removes it for developing. While the film is being processed, you X-ray the pelvis and hips, taking great care to move Nancy as little as possible.

Your first X-rays return and the new ones are taken out for developing. You put the X-rays on a viewing screen in the room. There are no problems with the X-rays, but Nancy definitely has problems. You can see on the screen what appears to be a skull fracture. She should be seen immediately by a doctor.

The hip and pelvis X-rays and a physician arrive at the same time. The doctor reviews the skull exam, while you check the other films for diagnostic quality. The doctor diagnosis a skull fracture. He quickly scans the other film. The hip and pelvis are broken too. This patient will be in the hospital for many long weeks. Chances are you will be seeing her again, watching her progress as confirmed by periodic X-ray examination.

The next few hours are extremely busy ones. Broken ribs, punctured lungs, more head injuries and fractures—the number of injured patients seems endless. But despite the pressure and growing fatigue, you keep working with the same accuracy and speed. By the time you have completed the last exam you have seen more than ten patients and really earned that long overdue lunch break. You won't be able to take a full hour, but even a short break now is welcome. You return to your department with the equipment, hang up your apron, and then head for the cafeteria. A short while later you are back on the floor.

The first exam is a special procedure, a lumbarmyelogram, where you will again be teamed with the radiologist. This exam, like many special procedures, requires the injection of a contrast dye into the patient, in this case into the spinal column. As in the GI series described earlier, the radiologist will watch the movement of the dye as it travels up the spinal column. If there are any defects or obstructions in the column, they will be observed.

You quickly prepare the examination table with sterile needles, syringe, and solution. You are careful to use sterile techniques to prevent any germ contamination. You measure the dye, assemble the needle and syringe, and then fill the syringe with the contrast medium.

Your patient, Mr. Demetrious, is very apprehensive about the exam. While you are draping him you carefully explain the entire procedure. You emphasize that an injection in the lumbar area is no more painful than a routine shot, and you assure your patient that Dr. Copeland is a pro when it comes to giving injections of any kind. He relaxes a bit. You cleanse the injection area with antiseptic. Dr. Copeland takes over from there. While you hold Mr. Demetrious steady, she palpates the area and finds the right injection spot. Then slowly the needle is inserted and the dye is injected. As it travels up the spinal column she observes the dye's movement on the fluoroscopy screen.

You carefully watch Mr. Demetrious for any rection to the dye. The exam goes well. No problems. This is your last "official" examination for the day. You are spending the rest of the afternoon in the CAT unit. You have been selected by the chief radiologic technologist to receive additional training, on-the-job, in this specialized area. Eventually, after training is completed, you will be permanently assigned to this area and work exclusively with the CAT scanner.

We will leave the radiologic technologist here, but will you leave this profession here? The choice is yours. If the radiologic technologist's job seems interesting and the work worthwhile, perhaps this is the profession for you. Perhaps this is where you might find your career satisfaction.

PERSONAL QUALIFICATIONS AND WORKING CONDITIONS

Seeing what the radiologic technologist does on the job should give you a good clue as to what special personal qualifications are necessary for this profession. The radiologic technologist must have:

- An ability to organize and analyze information (needed for determining the correct radiographic procedures to be performed and organizing daily work schedules).

- An ability to work rapidly and accurately, occasionally under stress.

- Good powers of observation and attention to detail (needed for observing patients' reactions and for performing radiographic procedures without error).

- Adaptability (needed for modifying radiographic techniques to suit the patient's particular needs).

- Basic communications skills (needed for communicating with patients, patient's families, and physicians; also needed for handling general clerical and administrative work within the unit).

Beyond these basic qualifications the radiologic technologist must be able to work well with patients of all kinds.

In considering radiologic technology as a career, you may wonder about the hazards involved and long-term radiation. Radiation is a two-edged sword that can help or harm. However, this no longer should be a drawback for anyone interested in this field. Radiation safety for both the technologist and the patient is a top priority of every radiologic technology department. On the job, radiologic technologists are protected by lead aprons, lead windows, and other safety measures which reduce or eliminate radiation exposure. Also, new equipment is constantly being developed which not only emphasizes improved diagnostic measures, but also minimizes radiation.

The profession requires active physical involvement with the patient. This means lifting, standing, moving, and positioning patients who often cannot help themselves. A knowledge of body mechanics rather than sheer physical strength is required for this, and women as well as men are equally suited for the profession. Work in clinics and private offices generally follows a 9-to-5 routine. In hospitals the X-ray department must operate 24 hours a day, so technologists must be prepared to work rotating shifts, including evening, weekend, and holiday work.

PREPARING FOR TRAINING

High school courses in chemistry, physics, and biology are important, since these are the basic disciplines upon which radiologic technology is built. Math skills, particularly algebra and geometry, are also needed in order to perform the basic radiologic equations. Though not required, typing is recommended because it makes the X-ray recordkeeping easier.

PROFESSIONAL TRAINING

If radiologic technology interests you, you can train for this profession in one of three ways: a two-year hospital school program, a two-year college degree program, or a four-year college degree program. All three programs emphasize the same basic radiologic technology curriculum; however, the two- and four-year college programs will also include general college work.

Your radiologic technology curriculum will include courses in physics, darkroom chemistry and techniques, basic principles of radiologic exposure, and radiographic positioning. Special training is given in the use of contrast media, radiation detection, and equipment maintenance. Anatomy and physiology are studied, and a general survey of medical and surgical diseases is included, since these subjects must be thoroughly understood in order to produce a quality radiograph.

Some basic training is given in radiation therapy and nuclear medicine techniques. However, these are now considered separate professions and a radiologic technologist does not generally work in these areas.

The special procedures described earlier are only briefly covered in the basic radiologic curriculum. Technologists who work in these areas are usually hand-picked by the chief technologist after demonstrating superior skills and ability. They then receive special on-the-job education and supervised experience until they are proficient in the new techniques.

Throughout the course there is heavy emphasis on gaining practical skills and experience, first by practicing on dummies and artificial arms and legs, and later advancing to working with patients under close supervision. Though the amount of practical experience will vary from program to program, it is recommended that each student perform at least 1500 examinations annually throughout his or her training. To obtain this much clinical experience, two summers of fulltime student work experience is usually required.

Which program you select will depend on your long- and short-term goals and your financial aid planning. In the past hospitals charged little or no tuition and frequently gave the student a stipend to help cover educational costs. Because of rising operating costs, many schools have been forced to abandon this procedure.

As a rule of thumb, though, hospital programs, overall, are less expensive than college programs.

In the long run, a college program offers the student the greatest chances for opportunities for employment, job advancement, and professional growth. Given equal experience, a student who holds a two-year associate degree or four-year bachelor's degree is more likely to advance to supervisory, teaching, and other high-salaried positions. College programs charge the same rates for a radiologic technology program as they do for their other college programs. In addition, students may have to purchase uniforms.

Most of the four-year bachelor programs in radiologic technology concentrate on liberal arts and science courses during the first two years. The final two years are devoted to radiologic technology studies. This four-year bachelor's degree should not be confused with an "advanced" bachelor's degree program offered by many institutions for graduate technologists who already hold an associate degree in their field.

Generally, programs are competitive and look for better-than-average students. Some hospital programs admit few students—as little as six—while others, particularly college programs, are much larger. In addition to a review of your high school record, a college entrance examination or standardized admission test may be required. Prior to acceptance, students must submit a statement of good health from their physician. They are routinely given a physical examination after they are admitted to the program.

PROFESSIONAL CREDENTIALS

After graduating from an AMA-approved education program in radiologic technology, whether it be a hospital or college program, technologists are eligible to take a national examination given by the American Registry of Radiologic Technologists (ARRT). Those who successfully complete the examination are designated as RT(R)(ARRT), which means they are registered technologists of ARRT. This credential is extremely important for future employment, since it attests to the basic minimum competency of the technologist. Most hospital employers will hire only registered technologists.

Three states—New York, New Jersey, and California—require technologists to hold a state license before they can work in that state. To qualify for licensure the technologist must pass a state examination. Several other states at the present time are considering enacting licensure programs.

JOB OPPORTUNITIES

The employment picture in radiologic technology is a changing one. In those parts of the country where there are heavy concentrations of basic radiologic technology programs, there are too many technologists. However, there are many areas of the country where radiologic technologists are in demand. The greatest demand, even in areas with a surplus of technologists, is for technologists who have superior skills, who can do special procedures or emergency work rather than just routine radiographic procedures.

Technologists versed in new technology, such as CAT scanning, will also be in demand. Ultrasound, which is discussed in another chapter, is also a new and evolving area which many radiologic technologists are learning through special on-the-job or formal education programs.

The majority of radiologic technologists are employed in hospitals, but clinics, private radiologists' offices, and industry hire technologists as well. Outside the traditional medical setting, jobs are varied. In a large industrial clinic a radiologic technologist may be on hand to provide routine examinations such as chest X-rays or immediate diagnosis of broken bones or other injuries. Industry also employs radiologic technologists for use in research and production. For example, X-rays can find flaws in construction and can examine the composition of materials. They can be used to measure the thicknesses of certain materials or to check quality control devices. Insurance companies employ radiologic technologists for use in their diagnostic screening programs. It is also not unusual to find radiologic technologists aboard large ocean liners, not as passengers but as working crew members providing basic services in the event of passenger injuries. Equipment manufacturers hire RT's as company representatives helping to keep hospitals, clinics, and other purchasers of equipment abreast of the latest developments in radiologic technology and processing.

Many graduates find their first jobs in the institutions where they were trained. Others use traditional employment services such as newspaper ads and employment agencies. The professional association, the American Society of Radiologic Technologists, also maintains an employment service which assists in placing technologists all over the country.

Starting salaries vary, depending on the employer and geographic area where you work; $10,000 to $11,000 is the general range.

THE REAL ATTRACTION

What turns people on to radiologic technology? The answers are as varied as the technologists themselves. This is how Joann Bradley, a radiologic technologist at Downstate Medical Center in New York, feels about her work: "In this field I know I am contributing to patient diagnosis and treatment. Without the information that I supply the physician, treatment cannot proceed. The doctor may know a bone is broken, but without the radiograph, he won't know exactly how that bone should best be set. There are times when the work may be routine, but patients never are. And with new technology constantly being introduced, I feel the sky's the limit with this profession."

For further information on careers, write:

American Society of Radiologic Technologists
55 East Jackson Boulevard
Chicago, IL 60604

For information on professional credentials, write:

American Registry of Radiologic Technologists
2600 Wayzata Boulevard
Minneapolis, MN 55405

CHAPTER III

The Healing Art

Cancer—it is perhaps the most feared word in the layman's medical language. And with good reason. Despite tremendous medical advances in conquering disease, cancer remains our number two killer, second only to cardiovascular disease.

Cancer plays no favorites. Men and women, young and old, rich and poor alike are among its victims. Each year about 385,000 people are counted among its death toll. But looking beyond those grim statistics, there is a hopeful side too.

More patients than ever before are being cured of cancer. In fact, two out of every six cancers, when discovered, can now be cured. And this ratio increases to 3:6 when cancer is discovered early. Even patients with cancers which were once considered hopeless, such as leukemia, are now, in some cases, being cured; in many other cases, long-term remission of the disease can be produced.

These changes, of course, have not happened overnight. They are the result of long years of work on the part of both research and treatment teams. Through the combined efforts of medical research scientists, physicians, nurses, and other allied health professionals, a diagnosis of cancer today no longer automatically means a death sentence.

Modern cancer therapy offers the oncologist, a physician specializing in cancer treatment and research, three major cancer fighting weapons: surgery, drugs—also called "chemotherapy"—and radiation therapy. Which treatment is used depends on many factors: the type of cancer the patient has, how extensive it is, where it is located, the physical condition of the patient, and the physician's own judgment. Sometimes only one form of treatment is used, but more commonly, today, they are used in one or more combinations.

Whenever radiation therapy is selected, as either partial or total treatment, radiation therapy technologists are there, directly involved in the cancer treatment. Just as the radiologic technologist uses X-rays and the nuclear medicine technologist uses radioactive substances to diagnose disease, the radiation therapy technologist uses both X-rays and other radiation to help cure or relieve the patient's symptoms.

As you might well imagine, this is a career where personal responsibility for the patient counts a great deal. The radiation therapy technologist's skills and knowledge play an essential role in the patient's fight against cancer.

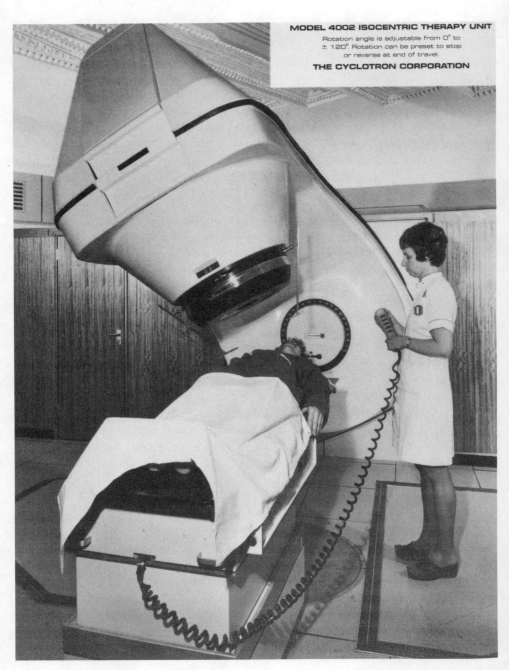

Radiation therapy technologist positions equipment prior to treatment. This machine, the latest in radiation therapy equipment, combines a cyclotron and a neutron therapy unit. Courtesy of the Cyclotron Corporation.

THE RADIATION THERAPY TECHNOLOGIST'S ROLE IN CANCER TREATMENT

About 80% of all cancer patients receive, at some point during their illness, radiation therapy. Consequently, technologists deal with patients suffering from almost every cancer type. Cancers of the skin, lip, oral cavity, lung, esophagus, cervix, prostate, colon, and brain are just a few areas where radiation treatment is used.

From the time each patient begins treatment, until it is over, the radiation therapy technologist is involved. During the course of radiation therapy, the radiotherapist, a physician who specializes in using X-rays and radioactive substances to treat patients, is responsible for the patient's overall care. But, unless the patient experiences an unusual problem, little of the patient's therapy time is spent directly with the physician. Most of the time, the radiation therapy technologist works with the patient, giving the radiation therapy treatment that has been prescribed by the physician.

Radiation therapy is based on the fact that "ionizing rays"—X-rays and rays given off by radioactive materials—are extremely powerful. They can penetrate almost all substances—rock, most metals, and human body tissues. When they are focused on and penetrate living cells, cell damage occurs. Just how much damage takes place depends on the strength of the rays and how far from the source of the rays the individual cells are.

When the atomic bombs were dropped on Hiroshima and Nagasaki, few persons died from the blast itself. Most were killed or injured as a result of the high radiation doses to which they were exposed. The farther they were from the area where the bomb was dropped, the lower their radiation injuries and death rate.

Today in cancer therapy, X-rays or other radiation doses which patients receive can be carefully controlled. The cancer cells themselves can be killed without totally destroying normal healthy tissues in the same area. In addition to cancer treatment, ionizing radiation can treat other conditions as well, such as a benign (harmless) tumor on the brain's pituitary gland.

Because each patient and each cancer is different, treatment dosages and plans for treatment vary. The exact dosage the patient will receive over the entire treatment program is determined by the radiotherapist. However, it is usually the radiation therapy technologist's responsibility to calculate the specific amount of treatment time necessary on a particular machine to administer proper treatment.

Before actual treatment begins, a great deal of preparation is involved. If it is the patient's first treatment, the radiation therapy technologist must first take an X-ray of the area which will be exposed to the radiation beam. This may be a simple X-ray or one which is more complex and requires the use of contrast media. A physician will then use this information to determine the exact area of treatment and treatment dosage.

Then additional steps are necessary. Many of these are similar to those which the radiologic technologist must perform before an X-ray picture can be taken. The radiation therapy technologist must make sure that the therapy machine is properly angled. The patient must be carefully positioned on the treatment table. (In some cases a treatment chair is also used.) The machine must be spaced at the correct distance from the patient, and only the treatment area must be exposed. Special filters or wedges which help to properly focus the radiation beam must be added to the machine, if necessary.

Finally, the patient must be immobilized. This is particularly important because, unlike an X-ray, radiation therapy treatment lasts several minutes. During this time it is important that the patient maintain exact positioning so only the cancer cells in the designated area are exposed to the radiation beam. Without the assistance of the various kinds of immobilizing devices, holding one position over a long period of time would be virtually impossible for many patients.

After each step in this process has been carefully performed, treatment can begin. Though all treatment takes place under the supervision of the radiotherapist, it is the radiation therapy technologist who works with the patient on a one-to-one basis, performing the treatment which has been prescribed by the doctor.

Because of the nature of their illnesses, some patients require special treatments. If so, the radiation therapy technologist may be required by the physician to develop a special treatment plan. Again, the radiotherapist will prescribe the dosage; however, it is often the technologist's responsibility to calculate the more specific factors which will be required for treatment. In addition to the factors which have just been described, the technologist must consider other variables. The specific direction of the therapy beam in relationship to critical parts of the body must be considered. The spinal cord or lungs, for example, are both easily damaged by radiation. A treatment plan must be devised which will radiate these areas as little as possible.

These calculations are complex and are usually made in the medical physics laboratory. They are commonly referred to as medical radiation dosimetry, which means the measurement of radiation doses for a particular patient. In some hospitals the radiation therapy technologist is responsible for these complex treatment plans. In other facilities these calculations may be done by a medical physicist.

But the complex, physical side of treatment is only one aspect of the radiation therapy technologist's job. During treatment the technologist works not only with the patient's body, but in a sense with the patient's mind. Throughout the course of treatment the radiation therapy technologist is in closest contact with the patient. An average treatment program will last from three to five weeks, and during this period four to five treatment sessions per week commonly take place. With this amount of contact, strong personal relationships develop.

The psychological aspects of this disease are as devastating as the physical. Consequently, the technologist becomes completely involved in the psychological as well as physical aspects of the patient. Most patients are frightened; their future is uncertain. From the beginning of treatment the technologist concentrates on relieving the patient's fears and building confidence as much as possible. This often means contact with the patient's family as well. They too, understandably, are anxious and upset. Their attitudes can do much to help or hurt the patient's progress.

Surprisingly, approximately 80% of the patients with which the technologist works are seen in the hospital radiation therapy department as outpatients. The remaining 20% are hospitalized for their illness. Many of these hospitalized patients are quite seriously ill. Treating them requires extra tender loving care. These patients are often at the lowest point in their lives, not only physically but also emotionally. With these patients the technologist's job often takes on an extra dimension. Simple nursing care procedures often become the technologist's responsibility. For example, a patient may be receiving oxygen or fluids intravenously (I.V., through the vein). In these instances the IV or oxygen tank must be periodically checked while the patient is in the treatment unit, to make sure that all is going properly. Some hospital departments have nurses stationed in a therapy unit who provide this care, but in many instances hospitals do not. This then becomes a part of the technologist's job.

The technologist must also be alert for any kind of patient reaction to treatment, whether it be breathing difficulties, shock, or even a cardiac arrest. Radiation treatment itself produces side effects in many patients, such as nausea or vomiting. If any problem occurs, the technologist must react immediately to comfort and care for the patient.

Throughout the course of treatment, the technologist must continuously assess the patient's overall physical condition. He or she must know not only when to give treatment but also when it must be withheld because the patient is too ill. For example, if treatment is administered when a patient's blood count is too low, the patient's immunological system (the body's natural defense system against disease) could be destroyed. This would leave the patient open to severe infections that could result from something as simple as a common cold. In this and similar circumstances, the physician must be notified immediately so appropriate medical treatment can be given and the course of treatment replanned.

As you can see, the technologist plays a major and important role in the patient's radiation therapy. But treatment involves the technologist in other responsibilities as well.

ADDITIONAL RESPONSIBILITIES

Wherever radiation is involved, recordkeeping is of vital importance. The patient's chart must document all aspects of patient treatment. This includes much more than simple identifying information and the equipment control settings; all information on the treatment itself must be included. Radiation doses that the patient receives during each treatment must be carefully logged. Because radiation doses are accumulative—that is, they build with each treatment session—the total amount of radiation the patient has received to date is recorded as well as the amount of radiation that remains to be given. This three-way check helps to insure that the patient receives the correct amount of radiation: not too much, which would be harmful and cause serious side effects, and not too little, which would leave cancer cells alive. Any patient reactions to treatment must also be carefully recorded.

Other aspects of patient treatment create additional responsibilities for the technologist. The technologists themselves make the molds which keep patients motionless during treatment. These molds cannot be ordered from a hospital supply company; each must be tailor-made for each individual patient. Technologists also cut lead into small, heavy blocks for placement inside the therapy machine. These blocks then act as shields which protect the patient's vital organs from exposure during treatment.

The equipment with which radiation therapy technologists work is complex. A fully equipped radiation therapy center at a major teaching hospital includes such sophisticated equipment as a six-million-electron-volt linear accelerator which produces very high-energy X-rays. This equipment is used mainly for very deep seated cancers. The department may also have a nine-thousand-curie telecobalt unit that can be used for stationary or for rotational therapy. Rotational therapy, during which the equipment rotates across the patient's body during treatment, is used when a cancerous tumor is located in a very difficult area to treat. Completing the list of high-energy units might be a betatron, which can emit a beam of electrons at any energy ranging up to twenty-two million electron volts. In the lower energy scales there will be X-ray machines operating on a kilovolt range and also diagnostic X-ray machines which can be used to locate and verify the tumor area.

Caring for this complex machinery is the responsibility of the biomedical equipment technician or the medical physicist. However, the technologist must be able to spot any equipment malfunction and, when it has been spotted, provide the biomedical equipment technician or physicist with specific information to pinpoint the exact problem. This requires a basic understanding of how each machine functions.

Completing the responsibilities of the radiation therapy technologist are activities related to simple department operations, such as patient scheduling and ordering supplies. Those technologists who are in advanced positions may be responsible for the overall supervision and administration of the department.

A DAY IN THE LIFE OF...

Unless you have been in a radiation therapy unit, it may be difficult to imagine working there. But if you can put yourself in this technologist's job for just a few minutes, you will experience a small slice of life in the radiation therapy unit.

It is still quiet in the radiation therapy department. Patients have not yet started to arrive. This is a good opportunity to review your patients' charts for the day. Today, indeed, will be busy and varied. Your first patient, a Mr. Curran, is being treated for skin cancer. He has been a sun worshiper all his life and, until recently, was totally unaware of the harmful effects of excessive suntanning. He is lucky, however. Skin cancer, especially when found early, has one of the highest cure rates of all cancer types.

His cancer appeared on his forehead as a flat, slightly raised cell growth. His cancer could be treated surgically; however, for cosmetic reasons, radiotherapy is the treatment of choice. Even with radiotherapy there are many ways this patient could receive treatment. Radioactive gold grains could be implanted into the tissues, or they could be arranged on adhesive felt and applied as a mold to the external surface of the tumor. In this case the radiotherapist has chosen X-ray as the treatment of choice for this patient.

Since Mr. Curran's tumor is small, less than five centimeters in diameter, it can be treated by a single exposure to X-ray. Since his tumor is also very superficial it can be treated with a lower energy X-ray dose. His tumor is located close to the eye, so a lead cut-out shield will be necessary to protect the delicate eye tissues, which are easily destroyed by radiation. When this patient's treatment plan was developed, the shape and size of the needed lead block shield, as well as the treatment area, were calculated.

You have already cut the block, which is matched to the contours of the area surrounding his treatment site. You carefully check the patient's record for the correct radiation dosages and then begin setting up the machine. You check the machine for the correct angle and radiation dosage and then gently position your patient under the X-ray beam. When all is ready, the lead block is added to the treatment tray that lies directly under the X-ray beam. Thus, when you apply X-rays to the patient, the lead block will shield the delicate eye area and only the area of the tumor will be treated with X-rays.

You explain the procedure to the patient and ask if he has any questions. You can tell he feels anxious about the treatment. The machinery is quite massive and frightening to him, as it is to many people. You explain that during the treatment you will be outside the room in the control area, but you will be observing him at all times. You caution him to remain motionless during the treatment until you return to the room. In a short while treatment is over and you are back chatting with Mr. Curran. He is feeling fine and did not experience any side effects as a result of the treatment. You explain that there will be some radiation reaction later, but that this is normal. He should not be frightened. Initially, about twelve hours after treatment, the skin will produce a faint pink blush. This is caused by dilation of the little capillaries in the treatment area. After an hour or two, that will fade. Later the skin will turn red again and he may also have some slight swelling. You tell him to keep the area dry and open to air and suggest that he apply some bland, soothing lotion if he wishes. Since treatment for this kind of cancer usually involves a single exposure to radiation, you probably will not be seeing this patient again. You caution him to contact his physician immediately if any unusual reaction occurs.

Your next patient is a Japanese woman, a Ms. Kyoko Kikuoka, a breast cancer patient. From a clinical viewpoint her case is an interesting one. Breast cancer is highly unusual in oriental women. The reason why this is so is completely unknown. It is one of cancer's many mysteries. She has already undergone radical surgery of the left breast. Since the cancer was present in some of her lymph nodes, radiotherapy is being used as a follow-up to surgery.

You will be spending the next several hours working on this patient's case, since the radiotherapist has asked you to develop a complete treatment plan. The patient is still hospitalized and recovering from the surgery. Before she is discharged, her treatment plan must be developed. In the following weeks you will be seeing her regularly.

You first spend a few minutes getting acquainted with your patient. She appears very withdrawn. You can understand her depression. You discuss what her treatment will involve. During the next several weeks, you explain, you, she, and the doctor will work as a team helping her to get better. She asks if you have worked with any breast patients before. Did the radiation treatment cure their illness? This is a delicate question. What your patient is really asking is, "Will I get well?" You gently tell her that you have worked with many breast patients before, and a great many of them do recover. In fact, you tell her, an old patient, Mrs. Kehs, stopped by last week just to say hello. She has returned to her life 100%. She is now working part time, caring for her family, and even playing tennis. Your patient listens with great interest. You change the discussion from cancer to some of her interests as you walk together to the treatment room. Dr. Price, her radiotherapist, is already waiting.

You help the patient remove the top part of her gown, while Dr. Price examines the surgical site. It is covered with a light surgical dressing, which Dr. Price carefully removes. You notice Ms. Kikuoka is watching you, looking for your reaction to her red surgical scar. Your expression doesn't change. You are a professional. No matter how the scar appears to you, your reactions can't show. That would influence the patient's feelings about herself. It is healing nicely, Dr. Price says. You ask the patient to lie back so you can take an X-ray. This X-ray will be used by the physician to determine the exact area which will be treated. You carefully position the patient under the X-ray machine and take the X-ray. You then drape the patient so her chest is not exposed and take the X-ray for developing. When you return, the radiograph is placed on a lighted screen inside the treatment room. Dr. Price carefully reviews it. He then makes a few marks on the patient's skin, which designate the general area to be treated. This is called the treatment field. He then writes a basic prescription for the patient's treatment. While he is seeing another patient, you will be developing the treatment plan based on his prescription. You carefully measure the size of the treatment field, which is expressed in centimeters (cm). In her case the treatment field is 10×8 cm, a total of 80 centimeters.

You will be using a teletherapy machine for this patient's treatment. This machine uses ^{60}Co, a radioisotope of cobalt that emits gamma rays, as its radiation source. Her prescription calls for 4500 rads to be given over a five-week period. A rad is a radiation measurement unit; it stands for *R*adiation *A*bsorbed *D*ose. This is the measurement of the energy absorbed by the cells from the radiation given. You must now calculate the number of treatment sessions per week and the number of minutes per treatment that will be needed to meet this patient's prescription.

Developing this treatment plan requires juggling many different factors. You will have to establish the tumor lethal dose (TLD), which is the dose of radiation high enough to destroy the cancer cells. At the same time, you cannot exceed the patient's tissue tolerance dose (TTD), which is the radiation dosage beyond which permanent damage to the healthy surrounding tissues would occur. The difference between these two points is the patient's therapeutic ratio.

But computing this ratio is only one factor. The kind of machine that is delivering the radiation also affects treatment. The higher the energy level, the more penetrating power of the radiation. The safety of the patient's healthy tissues is another important consideration. You must account for the scattering of radiation beams, a phenomenon similar to reflection. To compensate for this effect you will have to use certain wedges or filters. Even the size of the treatment field can affect your overall treatment plan. A large treatment field cannot tolerate as much radiation as a small treatment field. These are just a few of the factors which you must consider before you make your final calculations.

You help Ms. Kikuoka off the therapy table and ask her to wait in the hospital corridor outside. You explain that it will take you a while to develop the treatment plan, and it must then be reviewed by Dr. Price. She must wait because he has decided that today she will receive her first treatment.

You take the patient's chart to your office. Luckily you have a calculator, so you will not have to make these lengthy calculations by longhand. A half hour later you are finished. You have checked and double-checked your figures. You return to Ms. Kikuoka and accompany her to the treatment room. Dr. Price enters and reviews the treatment plan. It is satisfactory. Now the patient can be prepared for treatment. You take another X-ray film to make sure that the patient's position is correct for the treatment. This film is made using the radiation source of the treatment machine rather than X-rays, and using industrial-quality X-ray film. The results are not as high-quality as diagnostic X-rays, but are usable for this purpose.

Dr. Price checks the film and verifies by X-ray that the patient's treatment field and position are correct. Now, using semi-permanent ink, you carefully outline the entire treatment field on the patient's skin. This is a quality control measure to insure that only that particular area of the patient is irradiated. This is important for the patient's safety and it makes your job much easier. You also take a Polaroid picture of the patient with the treatment site exposed. This picture, which will be attached to Ms. Kikuoka's records, is another check to make sure the right patient receives the right treatment, should another technologist take over for some reason.

You then prepare your patient for her first treatment. You explain exactly what will happen during the treatment. She will feel nothing at all. During treatment she will not be on her back; she must be on her side with her shoulder back. This is not a difficult position to hold for a few seconds, but to hold this for several minutes requires some assistance. You gently move several sandbags to cushion her back and place one in front of her as an additional body support. You ask whether she is comfortable. When positioning her you must be very careful. Her left arm is still swollen as the result of her surgery. After setting the machine, you leave the room and head for the control panel, which is just outside. There, seated at a desk, you will be giving the patient treatment and monitoring her on a television screen. You will be able to talk to her by an intercom system. These precautions are necessary to avoid prolonged radiation exposure. Using the intercom, you talk to her encouragingly. You assure her that you are just outside and that you can, in fact, see her. "Please let me know immediately," you say, "if you feel sick. You don't have to be brave about this. I am here to help you." You ask her what the Japanese word for help is. "Pasuke," she replies. You both laugh as you try to repeat it. This helps relieve her tension. Treatment starts. Twenty minutes later, it is over. You reenter the room and move the sandbags, and help your patient sit up. She immediately complains of nausea. Her skin is pale and her respiration is shallow. You push her head gently down toward her knees. Just relax, you say. You quickly bring a basin in case your patient should vomit. In a few minutes the feeling passes. You take her pulse. Normal. Color has returned to her cheeks.

You explain the treatment schedule for the next few weeks and give her a few guidelines to help counteract her radiation sickness. Eat plenty of nourishing foods, you say, and cut down on roughage. As she returns to her patient floor, you begin carefully notating all the details of the treatment. You indicate the exact dosage she received during today's treatment and subtract this amount from the final total. You also indicate that she experienced nausea today. The physician will want to know this. If she experiences this again he may prescribe some medication.

The morning has gone quickly. It is lunchtime, so you return to your office. You are not going out today; instead, while you munch on a sandwich you will be working out some radiation dosimetry. This area of radiation therapy fascinates you. You would like to become more proficient in it. Though your radiation therapy training program did cover the basics of radiation dosimetry, you would like to build your skills in this area. Consequently, in your spare time you have been working with the medical physicist, assisting in developing complex treatment plans.

You pull your file on Mr. Cooper, a patient who has a tumor located deep in the chest cavity. Because of its location, his tumor is inoperable. An intensive radiation therapy program must be devised. Yesterday you met with Mr. Cooper and his physician and obtained the preliminary information needed to develop his treatment program. You had carefully measured not only his treatment field, but other portions of the patient's chest cavity. A mold of the patient's chest was taken so that you could obtain the contours of the patient's body. With this information, you are ready to start developing the treatment plan.

You take the first dimensions of his treatment field size and convert them into a line drawing on transparent paper. Next, the shaped mold is laid over the transparent paper so that the shape will correspond with the areas on your graph. Then the contour is drawn on the paper. When you are finished, you have a graphic representation of the patient and the tumor. Because his tumor is so deep, rotational therapy must be used. In this type of treatment the machine moves through a 360-degree arc instead of remaining in one place. This is necessary because of the high radiation dosages which will be administered to the patient. If only one position were used throughout treatment, not only would the cancer cells be killed, but healthy tissues would be destroyed as well by the high radiation doses. To avoid this, treatment is administered over a series of angles, using the tumor as a central pivot point.

Dr. Sedio joins you in your office. She is not an M.D. (Doctor of Medicine), but a Ph.D. in radiation physics. She carefully checks the calculations you have made. You then discuss the complexities of this patient's case.

After she leaves, you get ready for your last patient of the day. Mr. Moss and you are old friends by now. You have seen this patient several times over the last few months. He is suffering from lung cancer. There is no hope of a cure. His treatment is purely palliative. This treatment cannot cure the patient, but it will help relieve his symptoms. Over the last few months he has been in increasing pain and has been having difficulty breathing. The cancer, which hit his right lung and was surgically removed, has now metastasized, meaning it has spread to other parts of his body. A new tumor has just erupted in the area of his digestive tract. He is now receiving radiation to reduce the tumor, so that food can pass through the digestive area. Without this palliative treatment, the tumor will continue to grow and completely block the digestive tract. Unless he received nutrition intravenously, Mr. Moss would starve.

He is already waiting outside with his wife. In the last several months you have come to know her well, too. She always accompanies her husband for treatment. He moves slowly into the treatment area, in obvious pain. But he is a fighter and refuses to admit exactly how he is feeling. You know the last thing in the world he wants to hear is a "How are you feeling today," so instead you ask him about his favorite subject, sports. All the time he is talking about Jimmy Connors' latest tennis match, you are preparing him for treatment. Once the patient and the equipment are both ready, you leave the room to begin the treatment.

Mr. Moss continues to talk nonstop about the game. You notice he is becoming short of breath. You gently remind him to keep quiet and as still as possible during treatment. After the treatment is over you carefully notate the record, writing down the specific dosage to which he has just been exposed. Because he has been extremely short of breath, you feel Dr. Price should see this patient.

While Dr. Price evaluates Mr. Moss, his wife takes the opportunity to speak to you privately. She asks you how he is doing. She often asks you, rather than the doctor, questions about her husband's condition. She looks to you for answers because you have worked so closely with him throughout the course of his treatment. Besides, she feels shy about talking with the physician. With you she feels at ease. You explain that this treatment should make her husband a great deal more comfortable, and that soon he should be able to follow a normal diet. Mr. Moss comes out and joins his wife. You let them both know that they can call you any time they have a question or even just want to chat briefly. As they leave, you give Mrs. Moss' hand a short squeeze and tell her that you will see her in three days, when her husband is due for another treatment.

The rest of the afternoon will be spent in the mold room, fabricating a special neck mold for one of your patients who will receive radiotherapy treatment of the brain tomorrow. The neck mold will help to keep his head immobile during treatment. Before you can begin this, however, Dr. Price has asked that you prepare a radium dose which will be implanted into a patient to treat the cancer of her uterus from within. You know that since you will be working with radioactive materials directly, you must use extreme caution. In this instance you will load a small amount of radium into a special capsule which will then be inserted into the patient by the physician. Following this, she will be kept in a special area, isolated from the rest of the patients, because she literally will be radioactive. Nurses entering her room will wear protective shielding and anything the patient uses must be discarded. Even her waste products must be disposed of separately.

A short while later, your task here is completed. Then you are off to the mold room to fabricate immobilization devices to prepare for tomorrow's patients.

We will leave our radiation therapy technologist here, but what about you? Would you like to stop here, or would you like to know more about this field?

PERSONAL QUALIFICATIONS AND WORKING CONDITIONS

Radiation therapy technology definitely requires special people. While sensitivity and warmth are personal qualities necessary for any health professional who works directly with a patient, the radiation therapy technologist needs these attributes in extra measure. Other necessary qualities are:

- Good written and verbal communication skills (needed for keeping patients' records, explaining procedures to patients and their families, and also for working closely with physicians and medical physicists in developing treatment plans).

- An ability to analyze and coordinate information (needed to develop treatment plans).

- Organizational ability, adaptability, an eye for detail, and good powers of observation (needed for organizing and carrying out treatment programs, and for remaining alert to patient reactions and other problems).

Beyond these basic qualities, average manual dexterity and eye-hand coordination are needed.

The physical workday is demanding. For the most part, radiation therapy technologists are on their feet all day long. There is a great deal of physical involvement with the patients. They must be moved, lifted, and positioned. This requires moderate strength and a great deal of stamina. As one director of a radiation therapy program pointed out, this requirement is not necessarily correlated with weight and size. On staff at his hospital is a ninety-pound, five-foot dynamo who, by using her knowledge of body mechanics, has no problem working with patients.

Work hours themselves are fairly regular. Most technologists work a 9-to-5 or 8-to-4 workday, chiefly because the majority of patients seen are outpatients and these times are most convenient for treatment. Though the technologist may be on call, there is seldom an emergency in radiation therapy. Most treatment programs are carefully planned well in advance. One emergency possibility is when radiation therapy is required immediately following a kidney transplant operation in order to retard rejection of the new organ by the body. Another emergency situation occurs when the spontaneous and rapid growth of a cancerous tumor presses on the superior vena cava, a major blood vessel. Without radiation therapy treatment the tumor grows rapidly and uncontrollably, literally cutting off the patient's blood supply. This responds with equal rapidity to treatment. Within twenty-four hours, the fast-growing type of tumor can be destroyed by radiation. Both these situations, however, are uncommon, and in general technologists do not work evenings or nights.

Two concerns often voiced by persons considering this field are questions of radiation safety and the depressing nature of the work. While these are valid questions to ask, the answers may surprise you. This job is neither hazardous nor depressing.

All health professionals who work with radiation must be aware of not only the benefits but also its hazards, and radiation safety is a major concern of every therapy department. All technologists wear a special badge from the moment they enter the therapy department to when they leave at night. This badge measures the amount of radioactivity to which the worker has been exposed. This is carefully monitored by the medical physicist, and becomes part of a permanent radiation record. This log measures the technologist's radiation exposure not just during a work week, but throughout his or her entire employment lifetime. If the measurement begins to approach or exceed established safety levels, the technologist is immediately furloughed (usually with pay) from the job until his or her radiation level returns to within normal range.

As for the depressing nature of the work, this is a common misconception. Technologists interviewed repeatedly stated that though the public image of cancer may be one of hopelessness, they constantly see the bright side. As one student technologist said, "There is a lot that can be done to help cancer patients today, and I help to do it. Contrary to what most people think, a lot of our patients get well."

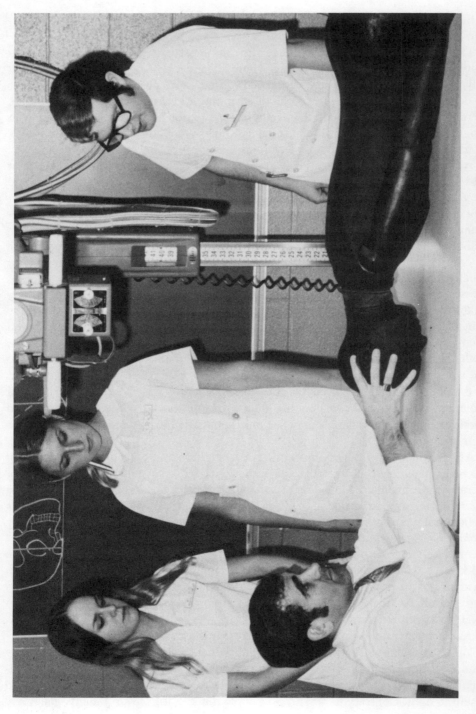

Students learn the basics of radiation therapy techniques by working with mannequins. Courtesy of Ohio State University.

PREPARING FOR TRAINING

Good high school preparation is important. Biology is a must because during professional training a lot of anatomy must be learned. Studying basic biology in high school makes this easier. Physics is important too. The principles of radiation therapy depend heavily on this basic science. Finally, basic math skills, including algebra, trigonometry, and geometry, are essential for computing percentages and dosages and developing treatment plans. On the job you will work with multiplication, exponents, and the inverse square law.

This doesn't require a math genius, but you must be reasonably proficient in this area. Many of the calculations are done with computers or calculators, but when these aids are unavailable, you must be prepared to make these calculations manually.

Because this is a people-oriented career, communications skills, particularly English, reading, and writing, will also prove useful. Psychology, sociology, and other courses that will expand your understanding of human nature are invaluable preparation for the training to come.

PROFESSIONAL TRAINING

Professional education for this career takes one or two years, depending on your previous education and experience. Two-year programs, which are given by hospitals, community colleges, and universities, admit students directly from high school.

All programs, whether hospital, community college, or university, offer the same basic curriculum in radiation therapy. The student receives the basic overview of physics, mathematics, anatomy, and physiology. Then these subjects are studied in relationship to radiation.

In radiation physics, the student learns about gamma, beta, alpha, and neutron radiation. The student is introduced to linear accelerators, the betatron, and the electron beam. The use of radioactive materials—radium, cobalt, and cesium—is also studied. Once the student understands the basics of radiation physics, this knowledge is applied to the human body: how the radiation affects both normal and cancerous tissues. Elementary pathology covering the normal and abnormal growth of cells is studied, as well as the various kinds of benign (harmless) and cancerous tumors.

With this as a base of knowledge, the student is ready to learn about treatment planning. Because the student frequently works with critically ill patients, basic nursing procedures must also be learned: how to take blood pressure, pulse, and respiration, obtain blood samples, assist with physical examinations, care for patients with radium implants, and the general care and precautions for patients receiving radioisotopes or other medication.

Radiation safety is another important part of the overall educational program, just as it is in radiologic technology and nuclear medicine. The radiation therapy student also learns basic techniques in both radiologic technology and nuclear medicine, since they are closely related to the therapy. Basic radiographic procedures are particularly important, since the radiation therapy technologist must know how to take a general X-ray of the treatment area before a treatment plan can be formulated. This does not require the expertise of a radiologic technologist, but it does require basic minimum competency.

Another extremely important part of training is clinical experience. Students are assigned a great deal of closely supervised work with patients. Though the amount of clinical work included in each program varies, about 2,000 hours is the average requirement. The two-year hospital program operates similarly to a hospital school of nursing and awards a certificate or diploma in radiation therapy upon graduation.

Community colleges award the associate degree upon graduation. Most of these programs are two years in length, but a few may run two and a half to three years. In addition to the radiation therapy curriculum that has been described, liberal arts courses are included.

Programs in universities are a recent development and are still few in number. They award a bachelor's degree upon completion and generally are arranged with two years of general liberal arts and science courses followed by two years of radiation therapy education. Thus, though the radiation therapy program itself is only two years, the entire program takes four years. In general, college programs, especially the bachelor's degree, offer the student the greatest opportunities for advancement within the field.

One-year programs are given principally by hospitals and cancer institutes and award a certificate upon completion. These programs follow the same radiation therapy curriculum already described, but they are more intensive and accelerated. For this reason, students entering these programs must already hold a bachelor's degree with a science background or a degree or diploma in registered nursing or radiologic technology.

Competition for admission is dependent upon the individual program. In general, most programs are extremely small, accepting anywhere between three and twelve students. A few college programs admit larger classes of twenty to thirty. Each year some program slots remain unfilled. The chief reason for this is that many students are unaware of the career opportunities which radiation therapy offers and they have a false impression of what this profession is actually like.

Admissions policies vary, but a transcript of high school or college work is always required. Generally, a personal interview and physical examination are also prerequisites. Some schools require that a student take a special entrance examination. Most hospitals charge little or no tuition, while college and university tuition rates are similar to other educational programs sponsored by the school.

PROFESSIONAL CREDENTIALS

Radiation therapy technologists are licensed in California, New York, and New Jersey. In order to qualify for licensure, technologists must pass a special state licensing examination before being permitted to work as radiation therapy technologists. In addition to licensure, a national examination in radiation therapy is offered by the American Registry of Radiologic Technologists. This exam, which is a rigorous three-hour written and oral examination, covers all aspects of the technologist's training. Upon successful completion of the exam, technologists may use the initials RT(T)(ARRT), which designates that they are registered radiation therapy technologists. Though this certification is not an employment must, it is definitely a strong asset, especially when one is seeking a supervisory or teaching position.

JOB OUTLOOK

At the present time there is a severe shortage of qualified radiation therapy technologists throughout the country. This trend is expected to continue for some time in the future. One reason for the shortage is that, in general, training programs are small. The number of therapists needed far exceed those currently being educated.

While the greatest number of job opportunities lie with hospitals, a number of radiation therapy technologists may also be employed by radiotherapists, physicians who specialize in the use of X-rays and ionizing radiation for the treatment of disease. In addition, job opportunities exist in research and teaching.

Industry offers the technologist a different employment option. Here, instead of working with patients, the technologist works with other technologists, acting as a sales representative bringing information on the latest equipment which has been developed.

Technologists working in hospitals are usually salaried. Starting salaries vary considerably, depending on the geographic area and the size of the individual institution; they range between $10,500 and $15,000. In a private office setting, technologists may also be salaried. However, individual radiotherapists may have other payment arrangements, such as profit-sharing.

WHERE YOU WANT TO BE

How does someone find his or her way into radiation therapy? Isn't it depressing? Bette Snyder, Educational Director of Memorial Sloan-Kettering Cancer Center's program, said, "I came from radiologic technology. I know I didn't want to be a nurse, so I got involved in X-ray. But then I used to wonder what happened to my patients after they left the X-ray department. That's where therapy is different. Now I get to know my patients, not just for a few minutes. I follow them right through their treatment. As for depressing, it really is a matter of viewpoint. I wouldn't call the job depressing, therapy is intense. It's really one of the most pleasant places to work. Here extra effort is taken to compensate for what the patients are going through. Instead of doom and gloom it is actually cheerful, especially when I see my patients getting better. Radiation therapy is where I want to be."

For additional information about radiation therapy, write:

> The American Society of Radiologic Technologists
> 55 East Jackson Boulevard
> Chicago, IL 60604

For information on professional credentials, write:

> American Registry of Radiologic Technologists
> 2600 Wayzata Boulevard
> Minneapolis, MN 55405

CHAPTER IV

The Nuclear Age of Medicine

On August 6, 1945, the earth stood still. On that infamous day the first atomic bomb was dropped on Hiroshima, a large Japanese city. Not even the expert scientists who had developed the bomb could predict the destruction and human misery which followed in the wake of that single act. Thousands in the immediate area of the bomb drop were instantly killed, and even those miles away from the blast were severely injured.

What caused such human devastation? Nuclear power. Today this energy force that snuffed out human life is being used to save it. Nuclear destruction has become nuclear medicine.

THE DAWN OF NUCLEAR MEDICINE

Though it was not until after World War II that any nuclear materials were available for large-scale industrial or scientific use, nuclear energy itself was not unknown. It had been discovered by Henri Becquerel in 1896, shortly after Roentgen's discovery of X-rays. Like Roentgen's, Becquerel's "discovery" came about accidentally. He found that natural sources of radioactivity existed—in this case uranium—as well as the electrically produced radioactive X-rays. However, it was not until the famous Polish scientist Marie Sklodowska Curie began studying these natural radiation sources that the first step toward nuclear medicine was taken. It was Madame Curie who coined the terms "radioactive" and "radioactivity" and who discovered radium, a radioactive element which is extensively used in medicine today. In addition to Madame Curie's contribution, other key discoveries paved the way.

Particularly important was the discovery of radioisotopes, atoms of the same chemical element, but differing atomic weights, which give off radiation; later it was discovered that these radioisotopes could be produced artificially. This final achievement led to basic experimental medical research with radioactive materials. Physicians and medical scientists learned that these isotopes could act as powerful tools to study human metabolism. Radioactive iodine, for example, yielded important information on thyroid function, and radioactive iron aided in the studying of iron reserves in red blood cells.

But the routine use of nuclear medicine to diagnose or treat illness was still

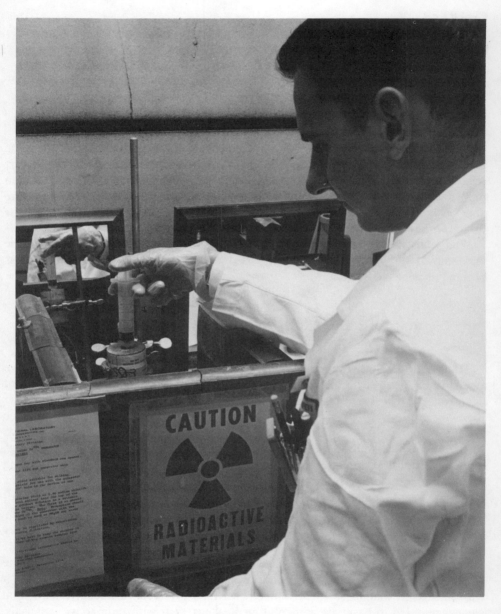

Radiation safety procedures are carefully followed by all nuclear medicine technologists. Courtesy of National Institutes of Health.

a dream away. Only a cyclotron could produce radioactive isotopes, and then only at great cost. The radioactive materials, or radionuclides as they are collectively called, produced via the cyclotron were not the best either. Many required considerable chemical manipulation before they could be used at all.

The development of the nuclear reactor in 1942 drastically changed this picture. But it was not until after World War II, in 1946, that even one nuclear reactor was available to create new radionuclides for other than military use. In 1946, the Atomic Energy Commission made a gift to the world when its "Manhattan Project" made radionuclides available for civilian use.

Today nuclear medicine is a widely used and invaluable tool which assists the physician in the treatment and diagnosis of illness. But nuclear medicine belongs not only to the doctor and patient. It is also the province of the nuclear medicine technologist.

MEET THE NUCLEAR MEDICINE TECHNOLOGIST

Who is the nuclear medicine technologist? A highly skilled health professional who assists the physican by actually performing the diagnostic tests and treatment procedures which require the use of radioactive materials.

Just as the radiologic technologist uses X-rays to produce a radiograph of the human body for diagnosis, the nuclear medicine technologist uses gamma rays, emitted by radioactive materials, to obtain diagnostic information.

The major difference between the two techniques lies in the source of the radiation. In the case of the radiologic technologist, an artificial source—X-rays, which are created by an X-ray machine—are applied to the patient's body. The nuclear medicine technologist, on the other hand, works with patients who themselves have literally become radioactive. These patients have received, either orally or by injection, carefully measured doses of radioactive materials (radiopharmaceuticals—radiodrugs) which have been specially prepared for use in the human body. These radiopharmaceuticals accumulate in specific body organs and tissues and emit gamma rays. Just as a prospector uses a Geiger counter to detect uranium deep within the earth by picking up the radiation it gives off, the nuclear medicine technologist uses special equipment to pick up and record the radiation which passes from the organs where the radioactive drugs are concentrated to outside the patient's body. This tells the physician what is happening on the inside. Though nuclear medicine may sound dangerous, in many cases the patient is exposed to lower radiation doses than with X-rays.

Sometimes the nuclear medicine technologist takes a simple measurement of the amount of radioactivity in the organ. But more often, pictures or images of the organs are made with the help of instruments called scanners or gamma ray cameras. The pictures produced by nuclear medicine techniques are different from

X-ray pictures. Where X-rays show different tissue densities, nuclear "scans" show the distribution of radioactivity within a given organ. They provide the physician with information about the organ's function, as well as its structure.

Not all diagnostic procedures are "in vivo," a nuclear medicine term which describes procedures involving the patient directly. Sometimes the nuclear medicine technologist mixes radioactive materials with samples from the patient, such as blood or urine. These "in vitro" procedures, as they are called, can detect the presence of hormones or drugs, or measure the amount of different chemical components of the urine or blood that are present.

The nuclear medicine technologist's jobs is not all diagnosis; there is a treatment side as well. You have already seen how the radiation therapy technologist uses X-rays and other radiation, such as radioactive radium, to help treat disease, primarily cancer. The nuclear medicine technologist also uses radiation to treat disease. Again, the chief difference between the two professions lies in the source of radiation. Radiation therapy technologists work with "closed" radiation sources. These are sources which are "contained," whether they are inside a machine and applied to the patient or implanted within the patient's body. Nuclear medicine technologists deal with "open" radiation sources. These radiodrugs are administered to the patient just as they are in diagnostic tests; however, a much higher amount is administered. Once inside the patient's body, they freely circulate until they accumulate in the diseased organ, where they kill cancer cells or combat other problems.

This is just a brief glimpse of how the nuclear medicine technologist is working with the physician. A closer look at the technologist's responsibilities will give you an even better picture of the important role they play in medicine today.

THE TECHNOLOGIST AND THE PATIENT

What kind of patient is a nuclear medicine technologist likely to encounter? Frequently, the seriously ill.

One important use of nuclear medicine today is to diagnose whether or not a patient's cancer has metastisized (spread) to other parts of the body. It is critical that the physician determine this before developing a treatment plan. If the cancer has spread, radically different treatment will be necessary. Once cancer treatment has started, nuclear medicine may also be used to periodically evaluate the effects of treatment.

Nuclear medicine does not diagnose only cancer problems. It helps to diagnose other conditions—strokes or blood clots and metabolism problems—and evaluate heart function. It can also help determine whether or not a tumor or a simple abcess is present in an organ. The brain, liver, bone, kidney, and thyroid are just a few areas of the body where nuclear medicine is valuable in diagnosis.

Close patient contact, both physical and mental, is definitely a part of this profession. On the physical side, to perform some nuclear medicine procedures, the exact anatomical area which will be scanned must be determined either by direct observation or with palpation (identifying the organ through touch). Like many other diagnostic techniques, the patient must also be carefully positioned. This definitely requires skill. Many nuclear medicine procedures take thirty minutes to an hour to perform. During that time the patient must be positioned not only for comfort, but in such a way that good diagnostic scanning can be obtained. Immobilization devices are frequently used to help maintain correct positioning.

In nuclear medicine, patient cooperation is essential. This is where the mental relationship between the technologist and patient comes in. To cooperate, patients must understand precisely what the procedure itself involves and how they can assist. Frequently this means talking not only with the patient, but also with his or her family. Physicians are usually too busy to explain these procedures in detail, so the nuclear medicine technologist fills this gap.

Like X-ray procedures, some nuclear medicine techniques require advance patient preparation. The nuclear medicine technologist often acts as a "patient instructor," outlining the specific routine which the patient must follow before the examination can be performed. Since families are involved in any illness, technologists frequently counsel the family as well on nuclear medicine techniques.

All work with patients does not focus on nuclear medicine. Sometimes simple nursing care becomes a part of the technologist's responsibilities. For example, patients who are seriously ill may be brought to the nuclear medicine department while they are still receiving fluid IV (intravenously, meaning through the vein). In this instance, the technologist monitors the IV periodically to make sure it does not become dislodged and that the fluid continues to flow properly. Though nuclear medicine procedures are painless and generally do not produce any ill effects, the patient's condition itself may require simple nursing care procedure. Liver disease often produces nausea in patients, so the technologist must be prepared in case the patient should vomit. When radiodrugs are administered by an injection, the technologist must follow good nursing techniques in preparing both the patient and the syringe for injection.

When performing nuclear medicine procedures, the technologist works under the physician's supervision. However, in most cases this supervision is indirect. The physician, usually a radiologist, prescribes the treatment or diagnostic procedure which will be performed, specifying the radiopharmaceutical, equipment, and nuclear medicine technique which are to be used. But the technologist takes over from there, calculating patient dosages, administering radiodrugs, and performing the examination. The radiologist is always on hand in case of emergencies; the technologist, however, performs the many nuclear medicine procedures alone or in cooperation with other technologists.

During the procedure, the technologist is completely responsible for the patient's care and well-being. The patient must be carefully monitored for any reactions to treatment or any physical distress from the condition being treated. During some procedures, the technologist works closely with the physician. For example, the physician may be administering a drug while the technologist may be recording important patient information, positioning the patient, or monitoring the equipment.

The duties of a nuclear medicine technologist do not stop with the patient. Like all health professionals working in medicine's new technology, the technologist has further responsibilities.

ADDITIONAL RESPONSIBILITIES

The technologist's additional responsibilities fall into three major areas: equipment, recordkeeping, and radiopharmaceuticals. The equipment with which nuclear medicine technologists work is among the most sophisticated in medical care today. In addition to using a Geiger counter especially designed for medical use to detect radiation, the technologist handles other special "scanning" equipment. The rectilinear scanner moves across the patient's body from side to side and up and down. It produces a line-by-line recording of radioactivity emitted by the patient. The gamma camera is used to record radiation over a specific single area or "field," or the patient's entire body, rather than a portion. Depending on the type of equipment used, the information that is picked up can be recorded either as a series of dots or slit-like marks on paper, or by a method which translates the radiation into a flash of light—a "scintillation" which can be recorded on paper or on an oscilloscope screen. The "picture" produced by these devices is actually a contour map which outlines the concentrations of radioactivity within the patient's body. This picture gives the physician the diagnostic information needed.

In carrying out nuclear medicine procedures, the equipment itself must be carefully positioned and focused. Special collimators may have to be used to adjust the focus of the area which will be scanned. The distance between the patient and the equipment must be fixed and the control settings must be carefully set so that the radiation can be properly detected. The recording mechanism must also be set and properly adjusted.

Just as the technologist monitors the patient during the treatment, the equipment must also be monitored for proper functioning. While the technologist is not expected to repair machine malfunctions, he or she must recognize when they occur. The technologist also helps prevent problems by operating the machine properly and following procedures to maintain it in good condition.

Throughout the technologist's workday, he or she is working with radioactive materials. The technologist calculates and prepares the necessary dosage of radiopharmaceuticals. This requires great care and precaution. Each technologist is responsible for radiation safety.

Recordkeeping in nuclear medicine is particularly important. An accurate log of all radiopharmaceuticals must be scrupulously kept. Results of the patient's examination must be carefully recorded. This includes not only patient-identifying information, but complete records of radiodrugs and their dosages, results of the examination, and any additional clinical observations. But before patient information can be recorded, the test results must be reviewed by the technologist, organized, and then presented to the physician. This requires some independent decision-making. After carefully evaluating the study, the technologist must decide whether or not extra measurements must be taken so that the physician will have a complete picture of the patient's condition.

The technologist's responsibilities are indeed varied. If you spend a short time inside the nuclear medicine department, you will see just how the nuclear medicine technologist puts radioisotopes into action.

ISOTOPES IN ACTION

The nuclear medicine department is already becoming busy and it is not even 9 o'clock. Today will be a hectic day. Not only are you seeing several patients, but you are scheduled to work this afternoon with a medical physicist in the isotope lab.

Before your first patient arrives, you do a careful equipment check. This is a basic part of the daily routine within the nuclear medicine department. First you test for background radiation in the area by adjusting your machine controls to the settings most frequently used. If the radiation count is unusually high, you will have to determine the reason. It may mean that your scanner is not functioning properly, or that a radiation spill has occurred somewhere in the area. But it's fine. So far there are no operational problems. You then begin calibrating your camera window. Throughout your equipment check you are noting all the information in your scanner log book. This record will help you evaluate the functioning of your equipment by comparing your results over a week, a month, and a year. Your scanners must always be in top working order. Your patients, the physicians, and you depend on it.

Your first patient, Ms. Lee, has just arrived. She is a tall, attractive young woman, but noticeably thin. Her problem? It is still unknown. It may be nothing. She is a dancer and leads an extremely active life. But her physician suspects it may not be her profession that has caused her sudden weight loss. He suspects an overactive thyroid may be the cause, a condition medically known as Graves' disease. Through you, her physician will soon know the answer.

Before you can begin your test, you must prepare the radiopharmaceutical. Because the thyroid gland has a tremendous attraction for iodine, it is a model organ for nuclear medicine studies. In fact, most of the original work done in nuclear medicine involved the thyroid gland. In this test you will use a radionuclide, a more precise term for these radioisotopes of iodine, ^{131}I.

You head for the "hot" lab, where all the radioactive materials are carefully stored far away from the patient area. Every time you enter this section, you are on the alert. Radioactive materials are serious business and deserve proper respect.

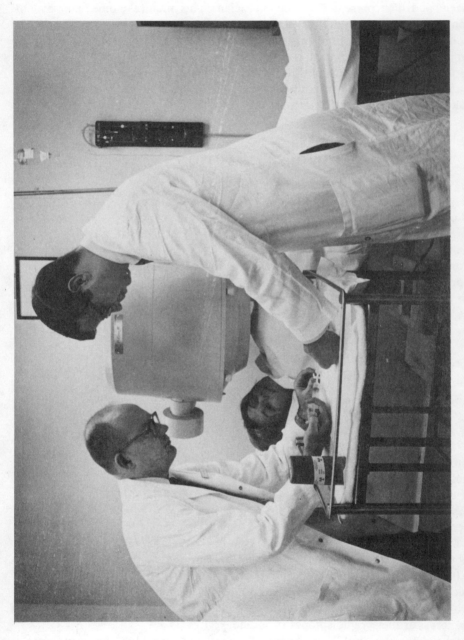

After the patient is positioned under the gamma scintillation camera, physician and nuclear medicine technologist prepare to inject radionuclide technetium 99. Courtesy of National Institutes of Health.

You remove the lead container marked "I" from the shelf, and note the amount and the date that are indicated on the label. Before you can make up the preparation for Ms. Lee, you must calculate its current strength. If this were regular or "stable" iodine, this information would not be important. Household iodine left on the shelf for days or weeks would be the same as when it first entered the container. Not so with ^{131}I. It has a half-life of 8.04 days, which means that in that time period half the material contained within would have decayed. One hundred millicuries, a unit of nuclear medicine measurement, of ^{131}I placed in the jar just one week ago would be almost half gone by now. One week from today another half of it would be gone. Because of this constant decaying process, you must calculate for this loss factor whenever you prepare a radiopharmaceutical. Each isotope has a particular half-life, which is noted on each bottle. You make the necessary calculations to complete the dosage. Before actually removing the iodine, you mix the special solution in which it will be diluted. Now you are ready for ^{131}I. Though you are working with a radioactive substance, you wear only light disposable gloves. The radiation to which you are being exposed right now is minor. It is similar to the amount of radiation to which you are exposed each day from cosmic radiation or radiation from the natural elements beneath the earth's crust. Even your own body has minute amounts of radioactive material, such as carbon 14. Lead-lined gloves here would be of little value. They would impair your ability to handle the containers and might cause a "spill," a far more serious problem than minute radiation exposure.

The three cardinal rules when working with radiation involve time, distance, and shielding. By working as quickly and efficiently as possible, you minimize the time to which you are exposed to radiation. Though you yourself are not encased in lead, all the radioactive materials in the lab are. You cautiously remove ^{131}I from its lead-lined container; measure the exact dosage; and pour it into the waiting solution. Then your "atomic cocktail" is carefully placed in a lead-lined container.

Ms. Lee has required no special preparation for this examination. All she must do now, you explain, is simply drink the cocktail. The ^{131}I will circulate through her body and move toward her thyroid gland. While this process is going on, you are getting ready for your scan, quickly and efficiently, observing the "time rule" in radiation. You position her on the examination table and set your controls, and minutes later your scan begins. A short while later you have your "picture." The thyroid gland looks like a large butterfly created by thousands of dots. Though Dr. Bacho, the radiologist, will interpret the scan, you can see from the image that Ms. Lee's physician was right. This patient definitely has a thyroid condition and will probably be returning to the lab some time in the future, for therapy. After she leaves, you finish recording your notes and review your next patient's record.

Mr. Kennat is a very sick man indeed. But you don't need a patient record to tell you that. One look at him makes that fact apparent. He has been brought down from his hospital floor and is sitting hunched in his wheelchair, a gray pallor to

his skin. He has cancer. Your role in his case will be to help determine whether
or not the cancer has already spread to his bone marrow.

You introduce yourself and carefully outline the procedure. He brightens a little
when you explain that scanning is painless. He has been through so much these
last few days and has been dreading another test. Just the words "nuclear medicine"
and "bone scan" sounded frightening to him. You make him comfortable while
you prepare your radiopharmaceutical—Technetium 99. Minutes later you return
to administer the dosage. In a bone scan this drug must be given intravenously. The
laws of your state and the policy of your hospital permit nuclear medicine technologists to do this. In some states, however, and in some hospitals, this specific
task is left to the physician.

You again speak reassuringly to Mr. Kennat. You will just feel a small sting,
you tell him. As you administer the drug, you watch Mr. Kennat for any reaction.
After the injection there will be a 15-minute waiting period to allow the drug to
permeate his entire body. Even though you will be working with a high-speed
gamma camera, this examination will take some time. In a bone scan, the entire
body is scanned, not just one bone. You will be required to make several different
images.

While you are waiting for the drug to take effect, you are busy. You are checking your equipment, taking a background radiation count, and logging information.
You are also chatting with Mr. Kennat, helping to keep his morale up.

The scan begins; almost 45 minutes later it is over. You now have a small
portfolio of images on this patient, half from scanning his body while he was on
his back, the other half from scanning him while he was on his stomach. After
Mr. Kennat leaves you will piece these together so that you will have a view of his
entire body. You will also mark the scans with prominent body landmarks, such as
his pelvic girdle, to orient Dr. Bacho when he reads the scans. Mr. Kennat is taken
back to his hospital floor by the aide, while you begin organizing the examination
results for the physician.

The rest of the morning goes quickly. An unconscious patient is brought down
for a brain scan and the cause of his unconsciousness, a blood clot, is discovered.
Another patient, Mrs. Scerbak, presents a particular challenge. She has been
hospitalized for a suspected pulmonary embolism, a possible blood clot in the
lung. This is very serious. If a clot is present and it moves, death would result
within minutes. This is one of the most technically demanding examinations. It requires a great deal of patient cooperation. In this particular case, the radionuclide
will be given neither orally nor by injection; the patient will actually inhale a radioactive gas. Because this examination involves her respiratory system, you have
already consulted with a respiratory therapist on suggested techniques. Before beginning the examination, you take time to explain in detail each step of the
examination and the part she will play. In the hot lab, you prepare the radionuclide
$Xenon_{133}$ for the procedure. You remove the container marked $Xenon_{133}$, note the
date and the amount, and carefully make your calculations.

The $Xenon_{133}$ is still in its liquid form. It is shipped in a simple saline (salt).

Using a large syringe, you draw in the proper dosage, and about 30 ccs of air as well. Then you shake the syringe and a chemical reaction occurs: the $Xenon_{133}$ separates from the saline solution into a gaseous state. You slip the syringe into a lead-lined container and return to Mrs. Scerbak. You now set up the spirometer, a special breathing device which will be used to administer the gas. You ask her if she is ready to begin the procedure and again you briefly outline each step. "Do you understand?" you ask. "Yes," she says. "Any questions?" you ask again. "No. I think I understand." You give her a reassuring squeeze and tell her just to relax and follow your instructions. You will be with her during the entire procedure. You put the spirometer mouthpiece and nose clips in place. Now she cannot breathe air from the outside. She is breathing only through the oxygen and carbon dioxide supply within the machine. You instruct her to breathe normally, and allow her time to get the "feel" of the machine. You ask her again if she is ready. She signals yes. Now you take your syringe and inject it right into the tubing. She is now inhaling not only oxygen and carbon dioxide, but also radioactive $Xenon_{133}$ itself.

You ask her to hold her breath immediately after she has exhaled completely. You then quickly take a scan. For the next five minutes she continues to breathe through the machine. You ask her periodically to stop and hold her breath while you take different scans.

Once the exam is completed, she cannot simply be removed from the machine. There is still radioactive gas within her lungs which, if expired, would contaminate the examination area. You explain to her that you will be removing the equipment shortly, but that she must exhale into a special bag so the radioactive gas can be trapped therein. There are many different bags which could be used, but your department has found that recycled weather balloons are ideal for this purpose. Before removing the spirometer and the nose clips, you have the bag ready and in place. You quickly remove the equipment and place the end of the balloon over her nose and mouth. She exhales into the bag and you quickly seal it. After your patient leaves it will be removed and eliminated in the outside air.

You finish notating the patient records and your scan and glance at the clock. It is hard to believe that it is already lunchtime. You are meeting Mr. Troughton, another nuclear medicine technologist, for lunch. He works in the "in vitro" lab. As often happens, your lunchtime conversation soon moves to shop talk. The work he performs is very similar to that of a medical technologist or a medical laboratory technician. This morning he has been working with blood and urine samples, determining the amount of radioactive materials present. One of the tests performed was for a man who weighed 400 pounds. The test he ran determined the amount of fat that was present in the body. His physician needed this information to develop a special reducing program which would insure exactly the right balance of nutrients to keep the patient healthy while he is on a literal "starvation" diet.

Another test he performed indirectly contributed to saving a human life. A car accident victim brought into the hospital had lost a great deal of blood; just how much had to be precisely determined. With a special radionuclide dilution test, the patient's blood volume could be calculated and the necessary whole-blood units administered. Though your friend has also worked with patients in the nuclear medicine laboratory, he prefers doing the "wet work" and now works solely in this area.

After lunch you head for the hot lab, where you will be spending the rest of the afternoon. A new shipment of radioactive materials is expected and you must carefully log in each item. Later you will be assisting Dr. Hitti produce radionuclides within the laboratory by a special process known as "milking." You will be working with radionuclide tellerium$_{132}$, the "parent," and removing (or milking) through a special nuclear process the "daughter" radionuclide, iodine$_{132}$, which has a half-life of 2.26 days. This milking process insures that radiodrugs are on hand. It also saves the cost of purchasing ready-made radionuclides. After this you will be able to call it a day. A very busy, but satisfying, day.

This technologist's day, as you have just seen, was indeed a full one. But was it one where you would find personal and professional satisfaction?

PERSONAL QUALIFICATIONS AND WORKING CONDITIONS

The qualities needed for success in nuclear medicine are similar to those required for radiologic technology and radiation therapy. Technologists should have:

- Basic communication skills (needed for working closely with patients, patients' families, physicians, medical physicists; preparing reports and recordkeeping as needed).

- An ability to organize and analyze information (needed for performing nuclear medicine procedures).

- Thoroughness, precision, and an eye for detail (needed, again, for nuclear medicine procedures; also for working with radioactive materials where great caution and care must be exercised).

Average manual dexterity for positioning patients and equipment is required. Because the nuclear medicine technologist works frequently with patients who are critically or terminally ill, nuclear medicine technologists must also possess that extra interest in and ability to work with people.

During the nuclear medicine technologist's day, he or she is extremely active: Lifting, moving, and positioning patients, positioning equipment, moving lead blocks and lead-lined isotope containers are but a few of the physical activities. Technologists also spend a great deal of time on their feet each day. Strength is not needed so much as stamina, good health, and a knowledge of body mechanics.

Nuclear medicine technologists must be concerned about radiation safety. They, like all health professionals working with radiation, are constantly monitored by a special radiation badge. The badge measures the amount of radiation exposure and insures that it does not exceed the basic safety standards set by the Atomic Energy Commission. As mentioned previously, many of the diagnostic tests performed with nuclear medicine actually expose both the patient and the technologist to less radiation than that of conventional X-ray techniques. So radiation exposure itself should not discourage anyone from considering this field.

The normal work day is seven to eight hours. A great many patients seen in the nuclear medicine department are outpatients; consequently, working hours correspond to their schedule. A normal work day might start somewhere between 7 and 9 A.M., lasting to between 3 and 5 P.M. In hospitals, there may occasionally be evening or emergency work, such as in the case of an accident involving a head trauma where an immediate brain scan might be necessary. When one is working for a physician, the work hours usually follow the physician's operating schedule, which is also designed around patient's convenience.

PREPARING FOR TRAINING

Because this is a science-oriented profession, students are advised to take science and math in their pre-professional years. Biology, physics, algebra, and trigonometry are courses which will prepare you for professional training. Courses which build communications skills, especially reading comprehension, are also useful, since student nuclear medicine technologists must be able to read and digest a great deal of medical and technical information.

PROFESSIONAL TRAINING

Nuclear medicine has undergone many changes. The first persons working in this field were trained on the job. Because nuclear medicine involves "imaging" and laboratory techniques, many of those first trained came from the ranks of radiologic technologists or medical technologists. Some also were registered nurses or persons (usually college graduates) with good science backgrounds. Slowly, as formal education developed, on-the-job training was discontinued. The first formal programs made a distinction between a "technologist"—a person trained at the bachelor's level or equivalent—and the "technician"—a person who had only two years' training. Today this distinction no longer exists, since it was found that both persons functioned equally well on the job irrespective of the length of the program.

Now, three separate training routes exist for the nuclear medicine technologist: a one-year program given primarily by hospitals and medical centers; two-year associate degree programs, and four-year bachelor degree programs.

The one-year program is designed for persons who have three to four years of college work with a heavy science background or are already qualified registered nurses, radiologic technologists, or medical technologists. Associate and bachelor degree programs admit students directly from high school. All programs follow the same fundamental curriculum in nuclear medicine technology, which focuses on six areas of study.

1) Physical science: the elementary aspects of the structure of matter, with special emphasis on the basis of radioactivity; radioactive decay; the interaction of radiation and matter; how radiation detectors work; and the basics of special electronic instruments such as amplifiers, scalers-rate meters, and computers.

2) Radiation biology and protection: the biologic effects of radiation exposure; the methods of reducing unnecessary radiation for patients, personnel, and in the general work environment; techniques to measure the levels of radioactive contamination, and various techniques of decontamination. Government regulations regarding exposure to radioactive materials and their proper handling are also an integral part of learning radiation protection.

3) Radiopharmaceuticals: how radionuclides are produced by reactors and by particle accelerators; how to formulate and prepare various radiopharmaceuticals in the nuclear medicine laboratory; how to establish and follow quality control procedure to insure the purity, sterility, and safety of all radiodrugs; and, finally, how these radiodrugs work inside the body.

4) "In vivo" procedures: the basics of using radioactive drugs with patients, including the operation of imaging devices with specific areas of the body such as the brain, thyroid, lung, heart, liver, spleen and other organ systems, and the use of different methods for time studies, such as computing cardiac output or cerebral blood flow.

5) "In vitro" procedures: the hazards of working with toxic chemicals, infectious biologic materials, and radionuclides; proper handling and disposal of such materials; how to use common laboratory instruments including pipets, centrifuges, ph meters, calculators, and others; establishing quality controls within the laboratory to insure reliability of all tests.

6) Treatment use of radionuclides: how to apply radionuclides to treatment; dose ranges for each particular problem; proper techniques for calculating the necessary quantities of radiodrugs; special problems of patient care radiation safety and follow-up.

In addition to classroom studies in these areas, students receive plenty of supervised clinical experience, usually over 1700 hours of clinical training. Clinical experience includes rotation through all basic areas of nuclear medicine. This helps a student learn all techniques and provides an opportunity to perform them often enough so that he or she becomes proficient in each.

Competition for programs vary. Some programs, particularly hospital programs, may admit as few as four or five students, while those centered in universities and community colleges may have large classes, as many as 40.

Students entering the one-year hospital certificate program must have college courses in anatomy and physiology, basic physics and mathematics, medical terminology, general chemistry, psychology, sociology, oral and written communications, and medical ethics and law. Under unusual circumstances, some schools may allow students to complete some prerequisite courses during the course of their one-year nuclear medicine training. It is assumed that medical technologists, radiologic technologists, and registered nurses already have the necessary educational background. Therefore, they are not required to complete these specific course requirements.

Associate and baccalaureate degree programs which admit graduates from high school require students to have had a concentration in the sciences. At the associate degree level, the first year is devoted to liberal arts and science courses and the second and final year to nuclear medicine training. In the bachelor's degree program, the first two or three years are devoted to liberal arts and science courses and the remaining portion to nuclear medicine education.

Training costs vary, but hospital and community college programs are generally inexpensive. Some hospital programs may even charge no tuition and offer a small stipend to students to help cover educational costs.

PROFESSIONAL CREDENTIALS

The picture for professional credentials in nuclear medicine is a changing one. At the present time licensure exists only in two states—New Jersey and Florida—but is being considered in twelve others. In some states nuclear medicine technologists are included for licensure under the broad category of radiologic technology because of the development of the profession. However, nuclear medicine is clearly recognized now as a separate profession. Technologists, through their professional societies in each state, are working to see that it is treated as such.

Again, largely because of the manner in which the profession developed, three certifying groups exist for nuclear medicine technologists. Since some NMT's come from the ranks of radiologic technologists or medical technologists, each of their professional certifying groups, the American Registry of Radiologic Technologists and the Board of Registry of the American Society of Clinical Pathologists respectively, certify nuclear medicine technologists. In addition, the Nuclear Medicine Technology Certification Board, the newest certifying agency, provides nuclear medicine technologists the opportunity to test their formal knowledge in nuclear medicine by sitting for a special examination. Upon completing this examination they are not designated CNMT, Certified Nuclear Medical Technologists. Those technologists who opt for certification by the other registries are designated NMT(N)(ARRT) when certified by the American Registry of Radiologic Technologists and NM(ASCP) when certified by the Board of Registry of the American Society of Clinical Pathologists. At the present time, obtaining these professional credentials is purely voluntary. However, they are becoming increasingly more important in employment. Employers in states where there are no licensing requirements are looking to certification as a substitute to insure that technologists they hire are fully competent to provide nuclear medicine services.

As a technologist you will definitely want to obtain certification from one of these organizations. Since each certifying board is equally recognized by employers and professionals alike, certification from one is as acceptable as from another.

JOB OPPORTUNITIES

The nuclear medicine field is expanding rapidly. In 1975 there were 5,000 jobs available for nuclear medicine technologists. To fill the current need, more than 600 additional NMTs must be trained each year for at least the next five years. Though there has been an increase in training programs, this annual need for more technologists is not being met.

Nuclear medicine departments formerly were found only in large hospitals or medical centers. This is no longer true. Nuclear medicine departments are developing in smaller hospitals of between 50 and 100 beds because of the increasing recognition of the importance of nuclear medicine procedures. The Joint Commission on Accreditation of Hospitals, the organization which reviews the services provided by all hospitals, now requires all accredited hospitals to provide nuclear medicine services, either in the hospital or through convenient arrangements with other facilities. All patients must have access to these important procedures. Thus far, economic situations seem to have had little influence on the nuclear medicine field.

Though nuclear medicine is expanding, jobs are not evenly distributed throughout the country. Therefore, graduates must be prepared to go where the jobs are. Since nuclear medicine services and programs started in large hospitals, usually located in urban areas, the job market in those areas is generally well supplied with qualified nuclear medicine technologists. The greatest need for technologists is in the newly established NMT departments in smaller hospitals, which are located some distance from urban areas.

In addition to working in clinical facilities, nuclear medicine technologists may find employment opportunities in private physicians' offices, teaching institutions, and industry. Some NMTs may also work in administrative or research fields.

In the long run, education and experience are the keys to job advancement within the field. A bachelor's degree is particularly marketable. Frequently the additional expense incurred in obtaining this degree is returned in the form of faster promotions, job advancement, and increased salaries.

Starting salaries range between $9,000 and $13,000, depending on the geographic area, the professional education, and whether or not a technologist is certified. Salaries increase with advanced education and experience. Depending on the size of the hospital, a chief technologist may earn between $18,000 and $22,000.

First jobs are usually secured through newspaper ads, ads in professional journals, or by placement services offered through the schools. The professional organizations which represent nuclear medicine technologists have job placement services as well.

MEETING THE CHALLENGE

If you choose to work in the nuclear medicine health field, what should you expect? "New developments," says Sue Engelkes Levine, Educational Coordinator of New York University's Nuclear Medicine Technology Program. "Though some nuclear medicine procedures are routine, the field on the whole is an interesting and exciting one. Technologists today must face the challenge of constant changes. Computers have been added to nuclear medicine; many of the radioisotopes we are working with today were unknown just a few years ago. In nuclear medicine you also have a chance to pick an area where you fit in best, whether it is working with patients or in the laboratory. I may be prejudiced, but I would recommend nuclear medicine to anyone."

For additional information on nuclear medicine technology, write:

Society of Nuclear Medicine
475 Park Avenue South
New York, NY 10016

For information on professional credentials, write:

Nuclear Medicine Technology Certification Board
475 Park Avenue South
New York, NY 10016

American Registry of Radiologic Technologists
2600 Wayzata Boulevard
Minneapolis, MN 55405

Board of Registry
American Society of Clinical Pathologists
Post Office Box 4872
Chicago, IL 60612

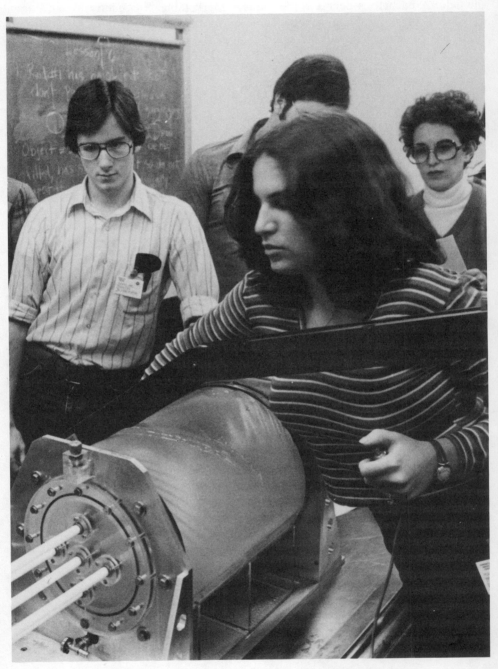

Student tries out basic skills in diagnostic medical sonography on a training tank which simulates the human midsection. Courtesy of Downstate Medical Center, State University of New York.

CHAPTER V

Seeing with Sound

What does a dolphin have to do with health care today? A great deal, and it can be summed up in a word—ultrasound.

Since its evolution, the dolphin has used high-frequency sound waves, ultrasound, to hunt its food supply and elude enemies. Now man, after years of research, is applying the same basic principle to probe the mysteries of the human body and to diagnose disease. These high-frequency waves can create body images which in turn tell us what's happening inside the human body. Ultrasound can detect gall stones, determine if a tumor is present, or tell if a mother is carrying twins long before the first heartbeat can be heard.

Though X-rays or other diagnostic techniques can do this too, the beauty of ultrasound is that it involves no risk to the patient. X-rays, for example, are a form of ionizing radiation and can cause genetic damage. Their use with expectant mothers can be dangerous, particularly in early pregnancy when they may cause serious birth defects in unborn infants. Ultrasound, on the other hand, has been used in hundreds of thousands of patient examinations—safely, without any harmful side effects. An ultrasound examination differs in another important respect. It is, to use a medical term, a completely non-invasive procedure. This is another reason for its safety. Unlike many other diagnostic examinations, no foreign substance has to be injected or ingested into the patient's body. This eliminates the possibility of a bad reaction or other accidents which sometimes occur when a foreign substance is used. Ultrasound has opened new horizons in medical diagnosis and created opportunities for a new breed of health care professional: the diagnostic medical sonographer.

In the simplest terms, the diagnostic medical sonographer is a specialist who uses ultrasound to visualize soft tissues of the body, such as the internal organs. But within this brief definition lies great knowledge, skill, and experience. To understand exactly what the sonographer does, you must first understand what ultrasound is and how it works.

WHAT IS ULTRASOUND?

Whenever we speak or a thunderbolt crashes or a dolphin transmits high-frequency waves through the seas, sound, a form of energy, is created. Sound is generated by the mechanical vibrations of the particles of the medium through which the sound waves travel.

Humans generally can pick up sounds that lie in the 16,000 to 20,000 Hz* range, but animals like the dolphin, bat, and dog can hear sound where human hearing stops. This is where the "silent" world of ultrasound begins.

Like all sound, ultrasound travels in waves. When these waves encounter a solid object, they bounce back and an echo is produced. The time it takes for the echoes to return, and their strength, provide information on the size, shape, and distance of the object encountered.

By using this echo system, the dolphin is able to locate a school of small fish for dinner; the bat is able to fly blind inside the cave, and the diagnostic medical sonographer is able to see what is happening inside the human body.

The first use of ultrasound was not in medical care but in warfare. Scientists, studying nature's built-in echo system, developed sonar, which was used during World Wars I and II to hunt enemy submarines. Afterward, other practical and peaceful uses for ultrasound were sought. Scientists soon saw a parallel between the submarine beneath the ocean and an unborn infant floating in a sea of amniotic fluid inside a mother's body. This theory was proved in practice, and obstetrics became one of the first major areas where ultrasound was applied to health care. Today, sonographers use ultrasound to provide physicians with diagnostic information in many other areas of medical care.

ULTRASOUND IN MEDICINE TODAY

While the sonographer may use his/her expertise in other areas of medicine, obstetrics is one of the major fields where ultrasound has proven invaluable.

As early as three weeks—long before any other tests perfected thus far can confirm pregnancy—ultrasound can detect fetal life. Though this would be impractical for general use, in some instances ruling out an early pregnancy can be critical; for example, where X-ray treatment or certain drugs may be under consideration for a patient.

Many of the other obstetrical exams performed by the sonographer are concerned with fetal growth and development. Since ultrasound has been perfected, a scientific table has been devised which matches fetal age with head size. Using this table, the ultrasound exam, and other patient information, it is possible to approximate the age of the fetus. Pinpointing fetal age is important in cases where abortion is being considered or an early Caesarian section is planned. The age of the fetus within just a few weeks can make a difference in whether the abortion can be safely performed or whether the fetus will survive the Caesarian section.

Ultrasound can also provide other information about whether the fetus is developing properly, is retarded, is suffering from certain birth defects, or has died inside

* Hz: Hertz, a scientific term for cycles per second.

the uterus. Certain diseases such as hypertension and diabetes can directly affect the unborn, so mothers with these conditions must be watched carefully throughout their pregnancies.

Ultrasound also assists in performing special obstetrical procedures like amniocentesis and fetal transfusions. Both these procedures involve entering a needle first through the abdominal wall and then through the placenta. Before either procedure can be attempted, the precise location of both the placenta and fetus must be known. This information is easily and accurately obtained through ultrasound.

Ultrasound is by no means limited to obstetrics. It is used in gynecology, where sonographers assist in identifying cysts, tumors, and fluid collection. Sonographers scan the abdomen to identify similar problems in the kidney, liver, pancreas, or other internal organs. Echoencephalography, the scanning of the brain with ultrasound, can pinpoint tumors or other masses. Echocardiography, the scanning of the heart, can be used to measure the functioning of heart valves and chambers. In ophthalmology, a sonogram of the eye can help to detect a detached retina or internal eye hemorrhaging. A special form of sonography, called Doppler sonography, can detect vascular problems, such as an aneurysm—a weakening and ballooning of the arterial wall, a potentially fatal problem when undetected. Doppler sonography also assists in monitoring fetal heartbeat and blood flow during pregnancy and labor. It also can detect kidney transplant rejection and detect air bubbles in the bloodstream.

The diagnostic uses for ultrasound keep growing with each new technological development. Its only limitations are those which govern sound itself. Sound is poorly conducted by solids and gas, so ultrasound cannot be used to diagnose skeletal problems or create images of gaseous parts of the body such as the intestines.

THE DIAGNOSTIC MEDICAL SONOGRAPHER AND THE PATIENT

Many sonographers work with ultrasound in all the areas just described. Some, however, specialize in one or more techniques, such as echocardiography.

While performing the examination, the sonographer works closely with the patient. Using a special device, a transducer, the sonographer can generate and direct high-frequency sound waves at the body area or organ which is to be screened. Because the human body is over 80% water, it is a good conductor for ultrasound. As the sound waves meet body tissue of varying densities, different echo patterns are bounced back to the transducer. These are then translated into a picture appearing on a nearby oscilloscope that resembles a small TV screen.

Where conventional X-rays give a frontal view of the body, the sonogram presents a cross-sectional or longitudinal picture. The image varies with the body area being "scanned" and the type of sonographic equipment being used. Some sonograms look like graphs and are similar to an EKG tracing, while others appear as shapes on the screen. The latest equipment can present images which are virtual "movies" of the internal body cavity.

Throughout the exam the patient, though bombarded with high-frequency waves, feels only a slight sensation of warmth generated by the sound waves and perhaps slight pressure as the transducer moves across the body. The exam is not only safe, it is totally painless.

These are the basics of the ultrasonic examination. Let's look now at the sonographer's other duties.

OTHER RESPONSIBILITIES

The sonographer's responsibilities do not end with the examination itself. Recordkeeping and equipment maintenance are additional duties that all sonographers perform. Research, teaching, and department administration may also be delegated to some sonographers.

Recordkeeping is extremely important, since the information obtained from the examination will be useful only if it is properly organized, recorded, and then presented to the physician. This process is more involved than the typical recordkeeping done for many other kinds of diagnostic exams. It is different because it requires some basic interpretation of the information.

As mentioned before, the sonogram doesn't show true anatomy; it shows a representation. This creates a situation which is very different from the physician diagnosing, for example, a broken bone by looking at a single X-ray. With the X-ray, the physician usually can clearly observe whether or not a break is present and reach a definite conclusion. Not so with a sonogram. A single sonogram, when viewed by itself after the examination, can often be open to various interpretations. The sonographer eliminates this margin for error by not only recording the specific details of the exam (e.g., patient's position, equipment settings, etc.) but by presenting a detailed account of what was seen during the exam. Sonographers also give their clinical impressions—that is, their basic interpretation of what they have observed. This information, coupled with the sonographs, gives the physician all he or she needs to make or confirm a diagnosis.

Depending on the policies of the individual sonography department, other recordkeeping may also be required. In many departments a running examination log is routinely kept. In the log each sonographer briefly notates each patient examination which is performed, and the results. Later, when the clinical results are definitely known, whether through biopsy, general surgery, autopsy, or birth, the log is checked. The actual clinical results are matched against the probable results as determined through ultrasound. For example, the fetal skull size as calculated by ultrasound will be matched against the actual size upon delivery of an infant. A cell mass which is removed through surgery will be checked against the log to see if sonography accurately diagnosed it as a tumor or a cyst. In this way, the log helps maintain and insure the overall quality of the exams the department performs as a whole, as well as those performed by individual sonographers. If the error rate exceeds the normal margin, the supervisor will want to find out where the problem is and correct it.

Equipment maintenance is usually minimal. However, the sonographer, like most health professionals who work with sophisticated technical equipment, must know how to operate the equipment efficiently and how to spot and correct minor equipment malfunction.

For the sonographer with superior skills and proficiency, there may be some basic research duties. Since sonography is an evolving area wherever it is being used, there are opportunities to develop and improve current techniques.

Finally, no department can function efficiently without overall administration. Many ultrasound units are placed in the radiology department, since ultrasound is an "imaging" technique. While the Chief of Radiology, a physician, may officially head the ultrasound department or section, the day-to-day operations are usually managed by the chief sonographer.

As you can see, the sonographer's responsibilities are varied.

What happens during a sonographer's typical day? Put yourself behind the scenes in the sonographer's place and find out.

BEHIND THE SCENES

It's morning, rush hour. While most people are hurrying to get to their office job, you are on your way to a large hospital not far from your home. You arrive shortly before 8 A.M. and don a white lab coat.

Your first patient is a young teenager, Ned Sanford, who has been hospitalized because his kidneys are not excreting urine properly. You review the patient's records and results of laboratory tests. Some of the chemical tests are within the normal range. Based on the results of these tests you suspect, as does his physician, that the kidney failure may be caused by an obstruction of some kind. A nurse's aide has already brought him down to the examination room.

You enter and smile. He appears ill at ease but relaxes when you call him by his first name. You explain the examination procedure and assure him that it is entirely painless. With that news his worried look completely disappears. You help him move to the examination table and instruct him to lie on his stomach. You expose the area to be examined and drape the patient. You first apply mineral oil over his body, which will assist in conducting the sound waves. Then you adjust the machine's controls and slowly begin to move the transducer arm across his body, moving first longitudinally and then transversely (across) the body.

All this time you are carefully watching the oscilloscope screen. During your preliminary scanning, you locate the kidneys and surrounding anatomy. You notice, in scanning the lower portion of the right kidney, that an abnormal echo pattern is reflected on the screen. This may be the obstruction. You take a series of Polaroid shots showing various aspects of the kidney. You're careful to take only those pictures which best visualize the anatomy.

It's just 30 minutes later. Your patient is surprised that the time went so quickly. You thoroughly wipe off the mineral oil and surprise Ned with a bonus for his cooperation—one of the Polaroid shots. You briefly explain what he sees on the photograph. He's duly impressed by the whole experience. The nurse's aide takes him back to his floor. You now sit down and carefully begin recording the details of the examination and your clinical impressions. After completing the information, you carefully file it in a holding file, where his physician will review it later in the day.

The next patient, Mrs. Kadunc, an outpatient, is waiting outside. You show her into the examination room and give her a hospital gown to change into. While she is changing, you review her examination form. She is decidedly pregnant, but the form, as often happens, doesn't indicate the particular reason for this obstetrical sonogram. When she is ready, you briefly question the patient. She explains that she is not due to give birth for a least another month. However, she and her husband would like to take a brief vacation before the birth of their child. Her physician wants to check the progress of her pregnancy to determine just how soon the birth may actually be.

Unlike an X-ray exam, where the patient's preparation frequently prohibits the drinking of fluid, this particular examination calls for a full bladder. When full, the bladder helps to push the uterus out from the pubic bone and also pushes the bowel away, acting as a "sonic" window allowing the pelvis to be more easily viewed.

You apply the mineral oil over the abdomen and pelvis, and then begin making a preliminary scan, moving your transducer in a longitudinal direction directly down the midline of the abdomen to the pubic bone. You then carefully move the transducer across her body, careful to maintain angles which are 90 degrees to the structures you are trying to see.

The placenta and fetus are easily located. You move the transducer repeatedly over the fetal area, determining which angles give you the best presentation of the fetus' skull. You move the transducer over the skull area and identify the midpoint of the skull by the different pattern it presents on the screen. This is the critical information which you need to calculate the fetus' head size, and in turn determine the baby's weight and potential maturity. You finish taking the necessary pictures, satisfied that you have all the information you need.

Mrs. Kadunc asks you what you can see on the screen and you point out to her the various structures: the bladder, umbilical cord, and the baby's head and body. She asks you if the sonogram can predict the sex of the child. Yes, you reply. Sonography, in some cases, can predict the baby's sex with fair accuracy, particularly in confirming a male if a scrotum-like structure can be identified. But, you add, second-guessing her, sex identification is only possible when the baby's position is just right. This is not the case with her baby today. The exam over, you

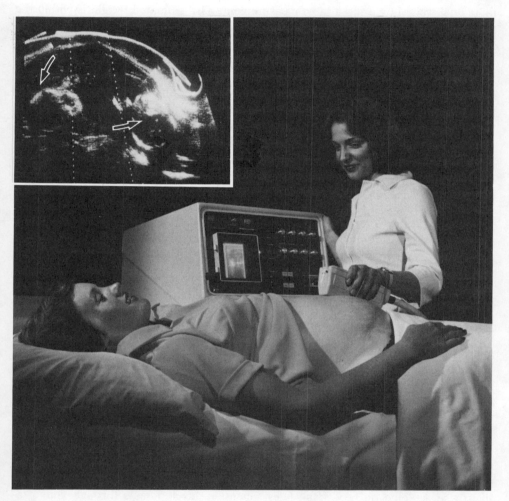

Sonographer performs ultrasound examination on obstetrical patient. Courtesy of Unirad Corporation. Inset shows sonogram of twins in utero. Arrows point to the heads of the fetuses. Courtesy of Maria V. Noifeld.

remove the oil and help her off the table. You instruct her to call her physician tomorrow. By then he will have the test results.

You carefully record all the pertinent information and calculate the actual skull size, compensating for the 40% reduction factor in the photo. You then approximate fetal weight by using a table measurement. The estimated weight is within the range of normal birth weight. Chances are, the doctor will veto any trip now. Birth could take place any day.

While you are finishing your notations, Dr. Ashley, chief of the department, enters the office and asks you to report immediately to the intensive care unit. Another sonographer will handle your patients until you return. She fills you in on the background of the patient you are going to examine. The patient, a middle-aged man, was admitted last night following a car accident. Though the initial skull X-rays are negative, his condition has deteriorated over the last few hours. The doctors suspect that a hematoma, a blood clot, may have formed on the brain. If so, surgery will be necessary in order to save this patient's life.

You gather your equipment and head for the patient's floor, reporting to the head nurse when you arrive. She briefs you on the patient's current condition and you quickly review the patient's chart. Your next stop is Mr. Martin's room. He is unconscious. You quickly prepare him for the examination, moving him as little as possible. You will be using the A mode scan, to determine whether or not a mass is forming on the left side of his brain.

You place the transducer next to his skull and quickly locate the midline of the patient's brain. You then obtain readings from the near and far sides of the skull and are ready to make your calculations. By comparing the difference in wave readings between one side of the skull to the midline and the other, you will be able to tell whether or not a hematoma has formed. If it has, the reading on the left side will be larger. The physician's suspicions are soon confirmed. The doctor in charge of the case enters the room. You present your clinical impressions. He reviews the reading, nods in agreement, and then leaves the room to schedule the necessary surgery.

You return to your department, where your next patient is already being seen by another sonographer. You use the time between patients to catch up on a little reading. Because sonography is so new and the field is changing so rapidly, it is essential that you spend time each week, whether at home or in "free" work periods like these, keeping on top of the latest scientific developments through your professional journals. Your latest edition contains a fascinating article which describes a new use for ultrasound—identifying various tumors by the kind of echoes which their tissues produce. Theoretically, the article summarizes, ultrasound will be used at some time in the future to make sonic biopsies.* These biopsies will identify whether tissue is cancerous or benign (non-cancerous) by a sonogram rather than surgery. Though the technique is only experimental, it sounds very promising.

---

* Biopsy: surgical removal of small tissue sample for study.

Before you know it, your next patient, Mrs. Ross, is waiting in the examination room. She is a middle-aged woman who has been hospitalized for tests to determine the cause of vague abdominal complaints. Her exam, and others like it, present a particular challenge. Going into this examination you are not sure what you are looking for and not sure what abnormalities, if any, you will find. This exam requires more than your technical skill. It tests your knowledge of normal and abnormal anatomy, diseases, and other conditions which can affect the body's functioning. The physician who has scheduled this exam must rely on your expertise and ability to identify any clinically significant information during the exam.

You briefly question the patient about her complaints and past medical history, and then carefully review the results of her other hospital tests, including her X-rays, nuclear medical scan, and laboratory workup. You are looking for clues which will help you decide on which areas you should concentrate during the examination.

After preparing her for the examination, you scan slowly and deliberately over her entire abdominal cavity, constantly watching the oscilloscope screen. During this preliminary scanning you are locating and identifying Mrs. Ross' unique internal anatomy. Just as no two persons are identical in outward appearance, our internal anatomy has many normal variations as well. What you must determine, however, is whether any variation is normal or whether it represents a pathological condition.

As you identify major organs, you mark her abdomen with a soft pen. These "X's" are important landmarks which you will need to perform the more detailed scanning which will follow.

You start your detailed scanning by concentrating on one section of her abdomen at a time. An unusual pattern appears on the screen. Before reaching any conclusion about the picture, you carefully rescan the area, checking your technique and the machine. The pattern is still there. It is real, not an artifact (a false picture caused by faulty technique or machine distortion). You slightly change the patient's position, finding a better angle for viewing the area. You take several pictures of this area and then continue scanning the remaining abdominal section. Finally, the exam in over. It has taken almost an hour to perform this examination thoroughly.

Mrs. Ross returns to her hospital room and you to your office to record your information in detail. Just as you are finishing, her physician enters to discuss the case. You present your clinical impressions, noting the size of the mass and the level at which it was seen. Based on the type of echoes which were reflected, your final clinical impression is that the mass is a probable tumor on the pancreas. You also mention to her physician the results of the particular lab tests which may indicate a pancreatic tumor as well. The doctor carefully reviews the sonogram and asks you several other questions about the details of the exam. Problems of the pancreas can be difficult to detect but the ultrasound exam now seems to confirm this as a strong possibility.

You glance at your watch. It is hard to believe but it is already past your normal lunch hour. You quickly head for the cafeteria and join some of your friends for

lunch. Then it is back to the department. There is only one remaining exam scheduled today—an echocardiogram. Your cardiac patient is not quite a year old and is
waiting in the examination room with his mother. You are grateful that she can
be there and help with the exam, thanks to the hospital's new optional "rooming
in" policy.

This mother has been spending every spare moment with her child, including
nights. With the security of having his mother on hand, little Danny doesn't
appear frightened at all, but he eyes the equipment with great curiosity. You introduce yourself to Mrs. Mulligan, answer her questions, and then enlist her help with
the exam. She rubs the oil over his tiny chest while you set up your equipment.

Like many babies born with heart ailments, Danny is quite small for his age.
This echocardiogram will help to determine the extent of the heart abnormalities
with which he was born. With his mother's help, you position him and are ready
to start the exam. However, before you begin, you introduce Danny to your
assistant, CoCo, a colorful hand-puppet dragon who will hold the transducer during
the exam. His eyes light up. Sure enough—CoCo, as always, does an excellent job
of keeping tiny patients distracted.

The exam is soon over, and as Danny waves goodbye to CoCo, you begin
recording your information. Using the data you have obtained during your exam,
you calculate the child's cardiac output—that is, the amount of blood the heart is
able to pump during a given amount of time. This is one important key to the
physician about Danny's heart function. Before the end of the day, you are scheduled to meet with Danny's physician to discuss the exam results in detail. In the
meanwhile, you will be meeting with a manufacturer's representative in order to
evaluate some new equipment which is being considered for purchase by the
Sonography Department. You have already reviewed the literature which has been
sent, and you are ready with your questions.

After these two final meetings your day is complete, provided there are no
emergencies. You are "on call" tonight.

What is your reaction to a workday like this? Would you find it satisfying?
Sonography takes a special person. Could that special person be you?

PERSONAL QUALIFICATIONS AND WORKING CONDITIONS

To do their job well, diagnostic medical sonographers need special qualifications:

- An ability to analyze and coordinate information needed to make clinical
  impressions.

- An aptitude for working closely with the patients; depending on the nature
  of the exam, the sonographer spends an average of 20 to 60 minutes working alone with the patient.

- Good written and verbal communication skills (needed for patient record-keeping and maintaining department logs; explaining procedures to patients and their families; presenting information to physicians).

- Organizational ability (needed for handling daily work load and department administration as required).

- Eye-hand coordination to operate equipment.

In addition to these general abilities, the sonographer needs good perception of spatial relationships and an eye for detail. This is essential for sonogram interpreting, since the picture a sonographer views does not show true anatomy but rather a cross-section or longitudinal representation. The sonographer must be able to recognize the various organs of the body by their relationships to each other as well as being able to identify any abnormalities present.

Working conditions in the field are generally good. Many hospital services such as diagnostic radiology (X-ray) or respiratory therapy operate on a 24-hour basis. This usually means a changing daily work schedule which includes evenings and night work, alternative weekends, and holidays on a rotating basis. Diagnostic sonographers, however, usually work a 40-hour week with a daily operating schedule of 7:00 A.M. to 4:00 P.M. or 8:00 A.M. to 5:00 P.M. Of course, when emergencies occur, sonographers will be expected to remain at the hospital until they are no longer needed. They may also be "on call"—that is, they may be called at their homes and asked to report immediately and work until the crisis is over.

In other work settings, such as physicians' offices or clinics, a daytime work schedule generally applies.

Physical activities during the average patient day involves standing or sitting during the examinations. Some lifting, turning, or other positioning of patients may be required, but this can be accomplished by men and women of average physical strength.

PREPARING FOR PROFESSIONAL TRAINING

Competition for professional training is keen. At present there are only about 50 training programs in the country. All programs require that applicants be high school graduates or the equivalent. In addition, two years of college with an emphasis on biological sciences or two years of training in a related medical field such as nursing, radiologic technology, laboratory technology, or other allied health areas is required by many (but not all) programs.

In high school and college, courses in mathematics and science, especially chemistry, physics, and biology, are particularly helpful for a career in ultrasound. Biology and chemistry are important because these are the basic sciences upon which an understanding of both normal and abnormal body processes are based. Physics is needed to master the fundamentals of ultrasound, which is based upon the physical characteristics and nature of sound waves. In certain forms of sonography, such as echocardiography, basic math skills are used for computations such as calculating blood flow.

While these are the minimum requirements in most programs, because schools have an extremely limited enrollment (generally between two and six students), preference is usually given to the applicant with a superior educational background. Many of the students applying to programs have college degrees.

As new programs open, this admissions scene may change.

PROFESSIONAL TRAINING

In the past, ultrasound training was all on-the-job. Most persons trained were already working in hospitals, usually in the radiology department, as radiologic technologists. Now on-the-job training is virtually nonexistent. Formal education is a necessity.

Training in ultrasound takes one full year to complete.

Most programs are hospital-based; however, a few university programs and junior college programs do exist. College programs will take two to four years to complete, since they combine college studies as well.

In addition to these formal educational programs, some short-term seminars in ultrasound are available. However, only radiologic technologists or other health personnel working in similar areas are usually permitted to enroll.

Because this field is so new, guidelines for educational programs are currently in the process of being drawn up by the ultrasound profession in conjunction with the American Medical Association's Committee on Allied Health Education and Accreditation. These should be published in 1979. Anyone interested in this field should be cautious about enrolling in a commercial program unless it demonstrates that it provides in-depth clinical experience with *real* patients in a *real* clinical setting.

Despite a school's claim, the basic classroom education and the practicing of sonography on fellow students is of little or no value without this clinical experience. Upon graduation, employment prospects for those without clinical experience are extremely dim.

A good educational program will combine classroom instruction with practical clinical experience in hospitals under qualified supervision. The curriculum will include courses in professional ethics, anatomy and physiology, abnormal pathology and clinical medicine, medical terminology, the biological effects of ultrasound, ultrasound physics, positioning techniques and instrumentation, film interpretation, comparison of ultrasound with other diagnostic procedures, equipment maintenance, and department administration.

Some programs cover all basic ultrasound specialties (echoencephalography, echocardiography, abdominal ultrasound, etc.). A few offer training in only one or two areas.

Tuition will vary with the individual school. Community college and university-based programs will offer tuition rates comparable to other programs. In general, students must pay for tuition, textbooks, uniforms, and, if applicable, room and board.

Some hospital schools may charge no tuition and/or offer a small stipend during at least part of the educational program. Upon the completion of a community college or university program, an associate or baccalaureate degree is awarded. Most hospital schools award a certificate or diploma.

Because so few degree programs exist at present, it is difficult to evaluate the impact of a college degree program vs. a hospital-based program at this point. In general, though, it can be expected that ultrasonography will follow the pattern of other technical careers in medicine. In the long run a college degree in this field will provide the student with an educational foundation necessary for more rapid professional growth and advancement within the field.

PROFESSIONAL CREDENTIALS

Thus far, diagnostic medical sonographers are not licensed.

Sonographers who complete a one-year training program and meet other educational requirements may apply to sit for a written and practical exam. The written exam demands a thorough knowledge of physics, anatomy, physiology, pathology, medical ethics, and patient care. The practical examination covers equipment technique and includes oral questions. Upon successful completion of this examination, which is given by the American Registry of Diagnostic Medical Sonographers, the sonographer is known as an RDMS—Registered Diagnostic Medical Sonographer. At the present time this certification is entirely voluntary, and not required to obtain employment. It is, however, an important credential which states to potential employers that the sonographer meets the basic standards of the profession. In the future, as more sonographers are trained, this registration will become more important in getting a job and advancing within the profession.

JOB OPPORTUNITIES

At present, the job outlook in this field is excellent. The number of qualified sonographers cannot keep up with the current demand. This situation is not likely to change unless there is a dramatic increase in both the number of training programs available nationwide and the size of their enrollment.

Currently, approximately 2,000 sonographers are working in the field. It is projected that within the next two years an additional 5,000 to 6,000 will be needed. Ten-year projections according to the American Society of Ultrasound Technical Specialists indicate that 18,000 to 20,000 may be needed. Although some of these sonographers will come from the ranks of those already employed in the health field, there should be ample room for those not presently within the field.

Hospitals are and will continue to be the largest employer of diagnostic medical sonographers, as more hospitals throughout the country expand their radiologic departments to include diagnostic sonographic services. Opportunities for employment also exist in clinics and other health facilities.

Specialized physician practices such as obstetrics and gynecology, where sonography can be used as a basic diagnostic tool with a large percentage of patient cases, also offer employment.

Sonographers are also in demand in government hospitals of the Veterans Administration, U.S. Public Health Services, and Armed Forces, both in this country and abroad.

Industry needs graduate sonographers, particularly those with college degrees and good science backgrounds, to work as technical advisers in developing equipment and as representatives to sell ultrasound equipment.

Because this field is rapidly evolving, research and teaching are other areas of demand. Faculty positions in hospital and university schools will continue to be available to qualified sonographers who will work as supervisors, instructors, and directors of education.

No "hard" statistics are available in salaries. In general, salaries in ultrasound range between $9,000 and $25,000, with industry salaries somewhat higher. Individual earnings depend, of course, on the years of experience, the geographic area in which sonographers are working, and their specific employment slot.

THE BEST REWARD

Of course each person's reason for choosing a career is unique. Marveen Craig, president of the American Society of Ultrasound Technical Specialists, explains why she feels so many people are entering this field today: "To me the field is constantly changing and challenging. It's the newest, most exciting, dynamic role in patient care today. I feel more like a colleague with the doctors, since I share my information and knowledge in helping patients. It lets me work closely with people, something which I enjoy. During the patient examination I spend more time working on a one-to-one basis with the patient than many other health professionals."

These, it seems, are rather compelling reasons for choosing a career as a diagnostic medical sonographer.

For additional information about diagnostic medical sonography, write to:

American Society of Ultrasound Technical Specialists
Box 1976
University of Kansas Medical Center
Kansas City, KS 64103

For information about requirements for professional credentials, write:

The American Registry of Diagnostic Medical Sonographers
Division of Cardiology
Children's Hospital
Cincinnati, OH 45229

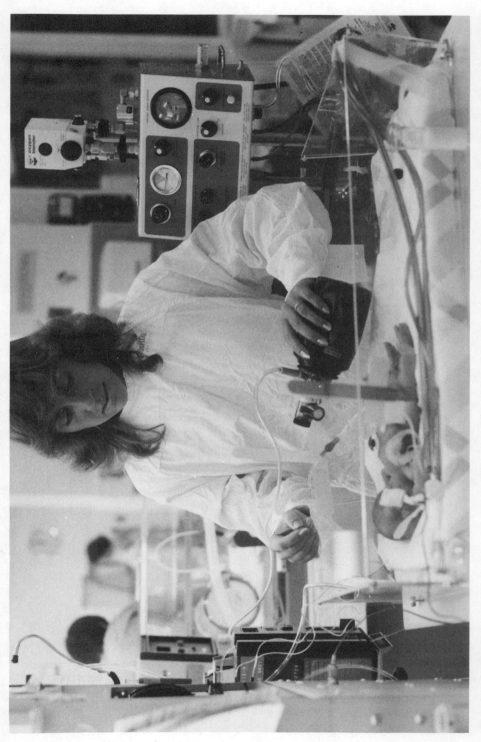

Respiratory therapist prepares to manually ventilate an infant who was born with immature lungs. Courtesy of Ohio State University.

CHAPTER VI

The Breath of Life

Have you ever swallowed a mouthful of food or water only to have it "go down the wrong way"? Or have you ever fallen and literally had the "wind knocked out of you"?

If these or similar situations have happened to you, then you have experienced, momentarily, that unpleasant and frightening feeling of not being able to breathe.

When your body's oxygen supply was cut off suddenly, without warning, your body signaled trouble immediately, and for a very good reason. Without oxygen you cannot survive.

You can live without food for a few weeks, and without water for a few days. But without oxygen, human brain tissues become permanently damaged within minutes, and after nine minutes the heart stops and death occurs.

Life-giving oxygen is brought to our bodies via the cardiopulmonary (heart-lung) system by a complex vital body process called respiration. Respiration is the foundation of the allied health science, respiratory therapy, and is the major responsibility of its specialists, the respiratory therapist and the respiratory therapy technician.

These specialists play an important role in health care today. With medical direction, these allied health specialists are involved in the evaluation, treatment, management, and care of patients with deficiencies and abnormalities of the cardiopulmonary system.

Their responsibilities also extend to teaching, recordkeeping, and equipment maintenance. Let's look at these areas in detail.

THE RESPIRATORY SPECIALIST AND THE PATIENT

The respiratory specialist's patients have wide-ranging problems from acute to chronic conditions. Some are the victims of hemorrhage, heart attack, drownings, electrocution; others suffer from lung cancer, emphysema, asthma, or pulmonary edema (fluid in the lungs). Whenever the breath of life is being challenged, the respiratory therapy specialist is called upon to intervene.

The respiratory therapist and respiratory therapy technician provide specialized and selected respiratory care to the respiratory distressed patient. This respiratory care has many facets.

73

Formerly the science was called "inhalation therapy," and its practitioners "inhalation therapists" and "inhalation therapy technicians." But as the profession grew, the name was changed from inhalation to respiratory in recognition of the fact that inhalation was just a small part of the overall treatment.

Perhaps the oldest and most familiar aspect of respiratory therapy is oxygen therapy. Immediately you probably envision an oxygen tent wherein a patient labors for breath. Advances in respiratory technology have made the oxygen tent virtually a thing of the past, but oxygen therapy, with modern equipment, remains a major form of respiratory therapy. Today gases other than oxygen, and medications, are administered to patients by inhalation. It has been found that some medications are best administered through the lungs as aerosols or sprays rather than by injection. This allows the drug to work locally in the lung areas as well as to diffuse through the body's circulatory system.

Aerosols and sprays are used not only for treatment, but for diagnosis as well. For example, a radioactive gas is administered to the patient via the respiratory system. As the gas is absorbed by the patient, various portions of the lung can be screened and evaluated for obstructions, restrictions, or other abnormalities. Other diagnostic respiratory techniques which are performed by the specialist might be the securing of lung secretions for cancer diagnosis or measuring lung volume and pressure to evaluate the effectiveness of the patient's pulmonary system.

Life support through the assistance of artificial airways, ventilators, and cardiopulmonary resuscitation is another major responsibility of respiratory therapists and technicians. Patients in the crisis situations mentioned earlier will all require intensive respiratory care and life support. Persons who have sustained multiple head or severe chest injuries (in car accidents, for example) usually require supportive mechanical ventilation (breathing). Through respiratory care and management, many who would have died are being saved and returning to useful life.

Respiratory care has preventive aspects. Respiratory treatment is often used prior to surgery. Breathing exercises and other respiratory techniques can help to clean the patient's lungs. This increases the patient's vital lung capacity and decreases the chance for surgical and post-operative complications.

The therapists' and technicians' work is indeed demanding and varied. In a single day they may see patients in the newborn nursery, surgical and medical wards, emergency, out-patient, and intensive care units of the hospital.

The equipment they must know and be able to use is as varied as their patients. Each patient's individual condition and particular problem dictates which apparatus can be used or what type of treatment given.

Respiratory therapy involves working not only directly with the patients, but also with other hospital personnel, particularly doctors and nurses.

The specialist always works to some degree with physician supervision. The chief of the Respiratory Service is frequently an anesthesiologist or a chest or thoracic physician.

Though the patient's physician prescribes a particular drug or respiratory treatment, it usually becomes the respiratory therapy specialist's responsibility to decide precisely how the drug or treatment will be administered and with what equipment. Respiratory therapy personnel, especially therapists, are frequently used as "sounding boards" by physicians. The doctor will discuss therapy with them and seek suggestions for in-depth respiratory management of their patients.

Because nurses are responsible for daily patient care, respiratory therapy personnel confer with them frequently to receive and transmit important patient information. Prior to performing respiratory therapy treatment, the specialist must have all up-to-the-minute information on the patient's condition that may change plans for treatment. The nurse in charge must also be informed that treatment is going to take place. Some respiratory treatment takes several hours; in these cases the respiratory therapist practitioner is usually not present the entire time and the nurse shares the responsibility of monitoring the patient.

During treatment, the respiratory specialist carefully observes and monitors the patient. Because respiratory treatment frequently alters a patient's physiological status, the specialist must be alert to any subtle changes or reactions which occur during or as a result of the treatment. Occasionally a reaction to medication may be severe, and the specialist must be ready to intervene promptly and minimize the danger to the patient.

THE SPECIALIST AS TEACHER

The respiratory therapy specialist is often involved in patient education and "in-service training." Many in-hospital respiratory treatments require the patient's cooperation to insure success. The patient who is under stress, who doesn't understand what is happening or why, will resist treatment. The therapist and technician must be able to clearly explain the steps in respiratory therapy treatment and gain the patient's willing participation. Patient education often involves not only the patient, but the patient's family, since continuing treatment frequently takes place in the home after hospital discharge. The patient and the family must be able to understand clearly not only the "whats" of continuing care, but the "whys," to insure that the prescribed program will be carried out.

In-service training, either in a classroom or at the patient's bedside, brings the respiratory and other hospital staff together. In-service training is a regular part of most hospitals' activities. It is a special education program which the hospital conducts to improve the knowledge and skill of its various personnel. In the case of respiratory therapy, this usually means teaching the nursing and resident physician staff. Because respiratory technology is advancing so rapidly, new equipment and procedures are constantly being introduced. These teaching sessions help staff keep abreast of changes. Instruction in good equipment safety practices and hygiene is also extremely important.

ADMINISTRATION

No patient care job, including the respiratory therapy specialist's, is complete without recordkeeping. A complete, clear, concise, and accurate record of the patient's management is essential if patients are to receive continuous and quality care. Hospitals operate a three-shift day. When the shift changes, the patient's record is the link which keeps the new staff informed of the patient's status and management. All respiratory treatments and procedures must be recorded and become a part of the patient's record. Such important information as the time, the type of treatment, medications given, patient's condition, attitude, and reaction to treatment, as well as any indications or contraindications for future treatment, must all be noted in the patient's record.

But the paperwork doesn't end here. Maintaining daily operations will entail keeping equipment maintenance records, inventories of therapy supplies, and department statistical records. Those in supervisory positions will have additional paperwork responsibilities, including personnel duties such as preparing department budgets, completing staff evaluations, and scheduling personnel for work.

MAINTAINING THE MACHINES

The respiratory therapist's and technician's job is not just with people. Machines and various respiratory apparatus are also an important part of the specialist's day. All equipment must be kept in top working order. A malfunction would not only prevent proper treatment, but could present a serious and even fatal hazard. Thorough familiarity with the equipment is essential. The specialist must not only know how to operate the equipment properly, but must be able to make minor on-the-spot repairs. Many substances specialists work with are potentially dangerous. Certain gases, especially oxygen, are highly flammable. Also, gas under high pressure can send loosened valves flying, endangering not only the patient, but the specialist and passersby as well.

Much of the equipment which is used must also be kept sterile. Disease can easily spread from one patient to another when using contaminated equipment. Proper aseptic techniques in the cleaning, sterilization, and utilization of equipment is as important as any other phase of the work.

You now have an overview of the respiratory therapy specialist's major responsibilities; is this a job for you? To help you get a real feel for this profession, try to picture yourself in the following situations which you might encounter in a day's work.

ALL IN A DAY'S WORK

"Code Blue, Code Blue" echoes over the speaker system, piercing the silence of the hospital corridor. Code Blue is the hospital signal for a life-and-death situation. From all parts of the hospital, people come running. The emergency cardiopulmonary arrest team assembles—the doctors, the nurses, and you, the respiratory therapist.

You arrive first at the patient's side. He appears limp and lifeless. With one hand you quickly feel one side of the neck and check the patient's pulse, while with the other hand you open the eyelids and observe the pupils. No pulse can be detected and the pupils are dilated. The patient is clinically dead (no signs of life) and actual biological death will soon occur unless you begin emergency medical treatment at once. You immediately start cardiopulmonary resuscitation, rhythmically pounding on the sternum of the patient's chest, artificially forcing the heart to pump blood. For every 15 beats you apply two breaths, via mouth-to-mouth respiration, to keep oxygen in the body's bloodstream. The rest of the team arrives. The physician now takes over the cardiac massage and orders medication, which the nurse begins to prepare. You move to the head of the bed and place an artificial airway in the patient's mouth, carefully twisting it until it is in the correct position. A hand resuscitator connected to a small oxygen tank has been brought into the room. You place the mask attached to the resuscitator over the patient's nose and mouth and squeeze the resuscitator bag gently, sending oxygen-rich gas into the patient's lungs. You check the pupils again and notice that they are starting to return to normal size. That's a good sign; there's probably no permanent brain damage. Within minutes the patient begins breathing on his own. The heartbeat has returned and the blood pressure is almost normal. You breathe a sigh of relief. A life has been saved. The patient is in stable condition and you are free to return to your daily patient rounds.

The first stop is a surgical ward where Mr. Wolfe, a heavy smoker, will be undergoing surgery in a few days. His patient record indicates that his physician wants the lungs as clean as possible before surgery. You instruct him in deep breathing exercises and coughing techniques and show him how to use a spirometer (a device which measures breathing capacity). You watch carefully as the patient follows your direction. Satisfied that he is doing the exercises correctly, you leave to see your next patient.

Mrs. Brown has been hospitalized for several days for intensive testing. As yet no diagnosis is confirmed. Her physician has ordered arterial blood gas studies. This will require you to draw an arterial blood sample, analyze it, and prepare the test results for interpretation by the physician.*

---

* This may sound more like a medical laboratory technologist's job, but remember, respiration is a complicated physical and *chemical* process and respiration in all its aspects is the respiratory therapy specialist's domain. This particular test yields information about the body's delicate acid-base balance, a part of the chemical chain of respiration. This tells the physician about the functioning of not only the lungs, but also the kidneys.

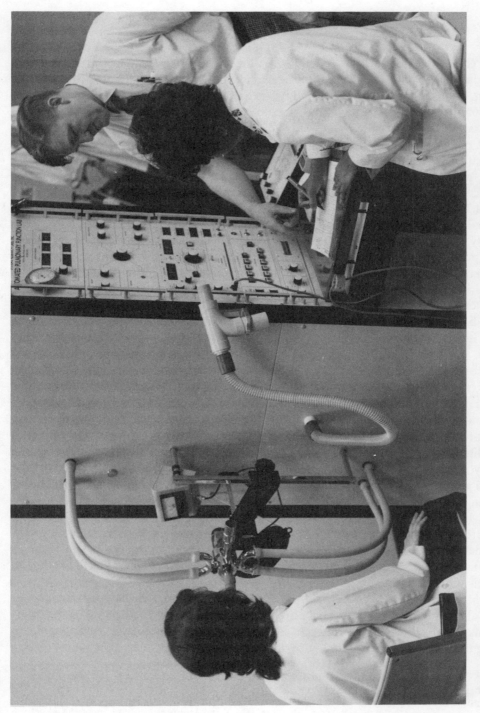

Using computerized analysis, lung mechanics are tested by a respiratory therapist. Courtesy of Ohio State University.

You notice that Mrs. Brown seems irritable—understandably so. She has already had several blood samples taken and doesn't welcome another needle. You explain the importance of the test and outline the procedure. The other samples that were drawn were venipunctures (taken from the vein). As the name implies, the arterial blood gas study requires blood from the artery. In this case the blood will be drawn from the radial artery, the artery which is usually felt when taking the pulse rate. Unlike the venipuncture procedure, obtaining blood from the artery will take several minutes, and Mrs. Brown's cooperation is essential. A careless puncture on your part or a sudden movement by the patient could damage the artery which is carrying oxygen-rich blood to the hand tissues below the puncture. Without an adequate oxygen supply these tissues would begin to die. You carefully palpate the puncture site and begin the procedure. In about six minutes you are on your way to the laboratory with the blood sample.

At the lab you calibrate the blood gas analyzer and run the sample through the machine. The lab report shows the pH level is on the acid side and the PCO_2 is below normal values. This could be an indication of diabetes. You discuss this possibility with Mrs. Brown's physician. Although the physician is responsible for making the actual diagnosis, he welcomes your interpretation of the test. Diabetes is a diagnosis he has been considering based on other tests, and the gas studies now confirm it.

A familiar sound is heard over the hospital's speaker system. It is your name being called, and you are being asked to report to Pediatrics. While it is not a Code Blue emergency situation, you move quickly, knowing that some problem exists.

In Pediatrics the nurse directs you to the "preemie" infants section. Inside an incubator is a tiny baby just a few days old, weighing less than three pounds. Born weeks too early, she must live in the incubator until her tiny lungs are fully developed and can sustain life. The nurse has called you because the oxygen level inside the isolette has risen dangerously close to 40%. Until recently, this hazard to newborns was unknown, but both you and the nurse realize that high oxygen levels can cause blindness in these infants. You spot the trouble—a loosened valve. With your wrench you quickly tighten it and adjust the oxygen gauge to the proper setting. In just a few seconds a problem has been corrected which could have caused a lifetime of heartache.

It's lunch break, and you go down to the hospital cafeteria. Today it's only a quick bite. There is still another patient scheduled this afternoon, and then an in-service teaching session. In less than a half hour you are back on the floor to see Mr. Veccio. He is having difficulty breathing because of a mucus buildup in the lungs. A few days ago he had major surgery and can't aspirate the mucus normally through coughing. Suctioning has been ordered by his physician to remove the obstruction.

Before giving treatment, you check the suctioning equipment and make sure it is functioning properly. With a stethoscope you listen to the upper and lower airways of the patient's lungs to determine which area is obstructed and must be suctioned. Suctioning is a delicate procedure and must be done carefully to avoid damage to internal tissues and bleeding.

You first use a hand resuscitator to get extra oxygen into Mr. Veccio's lungs. (Suctioning removes oxygen as well as mucus from the lungs.) Then you slowly insert a catheter (a tube) through the mouth past the larynx into the affected area. You turn the machine on and slowly begin to remove the catheter, rotating it between your fingers as it is withdrawn. You listen again to his lungs for signs of an obstruction. All clear. Mr. Veccio smiles. It's good to breathe easily again.

That's it for the day—with patients, anyway. You walk to the respiratory therapy department to have some time for yourself and prepare for the teaching session. This afternoon's group is a class of junior nursing students, and this will be their introduction to respiratory therapy. Your thoughts jump ahead to the rest of the day: review tomorrow's patient schedule; check current department supplies; inspect department ventilators for routine maintenance. Then home—it's been a busy day.

Were you able to see yourself in these situations, performing these jobs, helping patients with these problems? If so, perhaps respiratory therapy is a career you should consider.

THERAPIST VS. TECHNICIAN

Up to this point the term respiratory therapy specialist has been used to describe both the respiratory therapist and the respiratory technician. Both these professionals have the general responsibilities and perform the duties already discussed. You may well wonder, then, what is the difference between these two workers? The principal difference lies in the "hows," rather than the "whys," of respiratory therapy. The technician's training focuses primarily on the techniques, while the therapist's education has emphasized not only the techniques themselves, but the scientific theory underlying the therapy.

Technicians are prepared to handle the daily general respiratory care of patients and manage emergency situations as well. They function as "hands on" clinical practitioners. Therapists, however, have an added dimension. They understand the physiology of why something happens and can therefore exercise more judgment and accept greater responsibility in patient care. Patients with difficult respiratory problems or those requiring complicated procedures or intensive care are usually reserved for the therapist's management. Because therapists understand the fundamentals of respiratory knowledge, they are better equipped as potential teachers and supervisors of respiratory therapy. More frequently they will be called upon as consultants to physicians, to develop plans for patient care, and to coordinate therapy activities.

While these are the general distinctions between the two professionals, don't be misled into thinking the technician's job carries minimal responsibility. Local regulations and operating practices within the hospital determine which tasks each specialist will be expected or allowed to perform. Education, experience, and aptitude are also important determining factors.

Whether you opt for a career as a technician or a therapist will depend on your immediate and long-term goals, and your personal aptitudes and preferences. If teaching, research, and department management interest you, perhaps you should consider preparation as a therapist, since these are roles which the therapist is more likely to assume. If performing specific patient procedures and having daily patient contact give you satisfaction, then perhaps the technician's role is the one for you. Technicians, too, can advance to the therapist level with additional training.

No matter which role you select, you will be making a valuable contribution to the life and breath of the patients you serve.

PERSONAL QUALIFICATIONS AND WORKING CONDITIONS

What does it take to be a good respiratory therapy specialist? You may know the answer from what you have already read. The successful respiratory specialist will have several aptitudes:

- Manual dexterity and mechanical aptitude (needed to be able to operate, maintain, and repair respiratory apparatus).

- An ability to handle stress (needed to deal with emergency and other life-threatening situations).

- Good written and verbal communications skills (needed for working with patients' families and hospital staff, and for keeping patient records).

- Organizational ability (needed for managing daily work load and handling department administration as required).

Working conditions vary with each employer. Generally, however, hospital employment will require your working one of three eight-hour shifts, since respiratory therapy is a 24-hour-a-day service in a hospital. This means also that you usually will be working on a shift rotation basis with alternating weekends required. Specialists get a good deal of exercise during the day. They spend a lot of time on their feet, moving from one area to another, and patient treatment often involves standing. In the past, the size of oxygen and other gas tanks (300 to 400 pounds) limited the profession generally to men. However, this is no longer true. Equipment has been refined and tanks now are much smaller and lighter. But the specialist—male or female—should be able to move about 100 pounds, the weight of an average tank. Patients too must often be moved and positioned. This presents no problem for most women. In fact, about half of the respiratory specialists now employed are women.

PREPARING FOR PROFESSIONAL STUDY

Expect competition when applying to respiratory therapy schools. Although approximately 138 technician programs and 142 therapist programs exist, there are usually more students applying than there are program slots. A high school diploma or the equivalent is the minimum education required for admission to specialist programs. A good working knowledge of science and math is an essential foundation for respiratory therapy specialists. Respiratory therapy involves basic math problem-solving—an ability to use percentages, fractions, logarithms, exponents, and algebraic equations, and a knowledge of the English and metric systems of measuring. Calculus is not required but is helpful. An understanding of chemical and physical principles such as general gas laws, the states of matter, atomic theory, and the periodic table is also important. Computing medication dosages and calculating gas concentrations are just two examples of the need for science and math knowledge. Psychology and other social sciences will also be helpful, since respiratory therapy involves working closely with other people.

If you are weak in these areas, don't be discouraged. Concentrate on building these skills through a remediation program or refresher course. Remember, you do not have to be an outstanding student in these areas; you just must be reasonably proficient.

TRAINING FOR THE PROFESSION

This training is intensive (approximately one year for technicians, two years for therapists*) and includes classroom and clinical work.

The basic sciences (biology, chemistry, physics) and clinical sciences (anatomy, physiology, pharmacology, clinical medicine) are studied by both specialists. The therapist's course, however, is more extensive in both sciences and includes social sciences such as psychology, communication skills, and medical ethics as well. Both therapists and technicians must master technical skills: medical gas administration, humidification, aerosols, intermittent positive pressure breathing (I.P.P.B.), bronchopulmonary drainage and exercise, cardiopulmonary resuscitation, mechanical ventilation, airway management, pulmonary function study, blood gas analysis, and physiological monitoring of patients.

Programs for both therapists and technicians are offered by hospitals, colleges, and vocational-technical institutes. Those not given by hospitals directly will be associated with hospitals or other clinical facilities, so that students can receive

---

* There are some special one-year accelerated therapist programs designed for college graduates, registered nurses, or those who hold an associate degree in another allied health science.

the direct patient care experience that is an essential part of all health-profession training. Prior to admission most schools will require:

- a transcript of high school and college grades, if any;
- personal references;
- a physical examination (performed by your own physician or given by the school upon acceptance);
- completion of their admissions application form.

Entrance examinations may also be necessary. College programs may require the same admissions tests which all entering students complete (e.g., SAT or ACT). Other programs may use such tests as the California Achievement Test or the Allied Health Professions Aptitude Test. Some schools also require an interview after they determine that you meet their general admission standards. This will help them evaluate your maturity and real interest in the career. You should consider an interview even if it is not required. A good interview can be helpful in gaining admission to a program.

A program should be contacted as early as possible regarding its specific entrance requirements and application procedures. Costs vary tremendously, depending on the nature of the program. Some programs may charge regular college tuition rates while others, especially those given by hospitals, many charge little or no tuition.

The technician programs award a certificate or diploma upon completion, as do hospital therapist programs. Therapist programs given by two-year colleges and vocational-technical institutes usually award the associate degree. A few four-year colleges offer a baccalaureate degree in respiratory therapy.

PROFESSIONAL CREDENTIALS

The letters ARRT and CRTT are marks of distinction in the respiratory field. These distinctive professional credentials are awarded to those who successfully complete an examination in respiratory therapy. While these credentials are not generally required for employment, they testify to employers, patients, and health care professionals alike that you meet the highest standards of your field. Understandably, they are strong employment assets and an achievement you will want to attain if this is your lifetime profession.

Technicians are eligible to take the written examination, given by the National Board of Respiratory Therapy, after graduating from an American Medical Association (AMA) approved program and completing one year of work experience. If they pass, they are known as certified respiratory therapy technicians (CRTT).

The therapist examination has two parts, written and oral. Immediately after graduating from an AMA approved program, therapists (who have at least 62 college credits) may take the written examination. Graduates of two-year hospital programs must also meet this requirement. The oral portion can be taken once the written portion is passed and the therapist has had at least one year of work experience after graduation. This oral exam in particularly rigorous—only about 30% pass the first time. So therapists who complete both exam parts are very proud to be known as registered respiratory therapists, ARRT (American Registry of Respiratory Therapists), and to wear these letters after their names.

As of October 1975, 11,000 persons had been certified as respiratory therapy technicians and 3,077 individuals were registered respiratory therapists. In some cases persons held both credentials.

Two states, Arkansas and California, require respiratory therapists to hold a state license before being permitted to work. This is granted when one passes a state examination.

JOB OPPORTUNITIES

Respiratory therapy offers good employment opportunities as well as a choice of work settings. According to the Department of Labor, the employment of respiratory therapy specialists is expected to grow much faster than the average for all other occupations. One reason for this is the increased use of respiratory services within the hospital. A survey done by a Cleveland hospital shows that 25% of the patients entering the hospital receive respiratory therapy.

Many graduates find their first job through the school they attend, since employers, looking for respiratory therapy specialists, often go right to the source. Many students have found their first jobs by simply checking their school bulletin boards. The American Association for Respiratory Therapy, the professional association for the field, publishes job openings in its monthly newsletter. There are also job placement services which specialize in jobs for respiratory specialists. Graduates also use the traditional job-hunting routes such as contacting potential employers directly or checking with their local newspapers and professional publications where employers advertise.

Hospitals are the largest but by no means the only employer. Nursing homes, ambulatory or neighborhood care clinics, and rehabilitation and other health care facilities are all potential employers. Home care is another growing employment area. Here the specialist, like the visiting nurse, sees and administers respiratory care to patients in their own homes. This allows many patients, especially the chronic or terminally ill, to remain comfortably in their own homes rather than nursing homes or hospitals. Now that the hazards of air pollution have been clearly established, many public health and environmental organizations are employing respiratory therapy specialists. Colleges and hospitals also offer teaching and research opportunities, especially for the respiratory therapist. Private industry is another employer, offering positions in research related to new and improved product development and sales within the respiratory therapy field.

Salaries depend on many factors—experience, geographic location, size of employer, credentials. Starting salaries for therapists range from $9,000 to $11,000 with technicians' salaries about $1,000 to $1,500 a year lower.

WHAT MONEY CAN'T BUY

No matter what career you select, there are bound to be some aspects you will like and dislike about it. Respiratory therapy is no different. Not every day can be filled with the excitement of emergencies and the drama of saving lives. Therapist David Theuman of Bellevue Hospital, New York, tells it like it is when he says, "I like my job. I can see the results immediately whether I am doing a test, giving a treatment, performing resuscitation, whatever. Sure some parts are routine, and routine can be boring. But even when I am working with patients who I know can't be cured, I feel good because I am helping them make the best of what they have. I guess you could say I work at improving the quality of life."

For additional information about respiratory therapy, write to:

American Association for Respiratory Therapy
1720 Regal Row
Dallas, TX 75235

For information about requirements for professional credentials, write:

National Board for Respiratory Therapy
1900 West 47th Street, Suite 124
Shawnee Mission, KS 66205

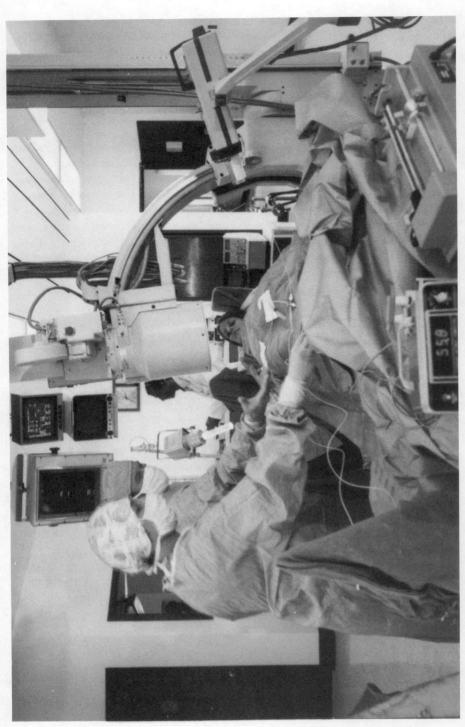

Physician and cardiopulmonary technologists prepare for cardiac catheterization. Courtesy of National Society of Cardiopulmonary Technologists, Inc.

CHAPTER VII

Double Duty

Your heart and lungs are your body's life support system, working together as a team to sustain life. In order to bring essential oxygen to your cells, each of these organs must depend on the other. The lungs take in oxygen and your heart, as your body's pumping system, circulates it throughout your body. Both organs are indeed amazing. In the course of the day your heart pumps about 5,000 gallons of blood, while your lungs inhale and exhale over 30,000 times. When the amazing work they perform slows down or is threatened by illness or injury, there is cause for alarm. The problem must be identified, evaluated, and treated if possible. Treatment and diagnosis are roles for the physician, but roles which they no longer carry out alone. Today they are assisted by many different health professionals, all working in cardiopulmonary technology—one of the newest and still evolving areas of health care.

MEET THE CARDIOPULMONARY SPECIALIST

What's in a name? In the cardiopulmonary field, a great deal. Because this field has advanced so rapidly, you will find a wide variety of occupational titles used to describe professionals working in cardiopulmonary technology. In addition, you will find a wide variety of professional duties to which they are assigned.

Cardiopulmonary technology is definitely in a state of transition. So before going any further into the roles and responsibilities of these important workers, a basic introduction to occupational terminology is in order.

Looking at the field most simply, technologists function in generally one of two major areas: cardiac or pulmonary technology. Some technologists work in both.

In cardiology technology, diagnostic tests now available to detect and evaluate heart problems have increased dramatically. Some professionals perform only one diagnostic cardiac test, while others perform several procedures. The job titles often used correspond to the test which the professional performs.

The most familiar test is probably the EKG, electrocardiogram—hence the most familiar job title, the EKG technician. But today cardiology technology includes far more than just this technique. New tests now include phonocardiography, a test

87

which picks up and identifies abnormal heart sounds and murmurs; vectorcardiography, a special recording of the heart's electrical activity; holter monitoring, a special 24-hour electrocardiogram test; stress testing, which records the heart action during physical activity, and echocardiography, which uses ultrasound to see the heart chambers and valves. (See also Chapter V, "Seeing with Sound.") Correspondingly, the people performing these tests might be referred to as the phonocardiograph, vector cardiograph, holter monitoring, stress testing, or echocardiograph technicians.

The tests just described are all medically classified as "non-invasive," meaning that during these tests no foreign object or substance enters the patient's body. In addition to these "non-invasive" tests, more complicated "invasive" tests are sometimes used to diagnose problems of the cardiovascular (heart and circulatory) system. During an invasive test, a foreign substance, such as a chemical dye, or foreign object, such as a tube, must enter the patient's body. For this reason, invasive techniques are considered more complex, and consequently there is an increased risk to the patient.

Technologists who perform invasive cardiac procedures are often referred to as cardiovascular technologists—or they may be known by the procedure itself. During a cardiac catheterization, a frequently performed invasive test, the physician, assisted by a cardiovascular or cardiac catheterization technologist, carefully inserts a catheter (tube) through the patient's vein into the heart in order to obtain special diagnostic information.

In the pulmonary area, the technologist is concerned primarily with diagnostic tests, both invasive and non-invasive, which detect lung disease or other respiratory problems. However, technologists may also perform respiratory treatment procedures as well. Pulmonary function technologist and physiologic technologist are just two titles often ascribed to these professionals. In many respects they are similar to respiratory therapists, since both work in the pulmonary field. However, the chief distinction between the two professions lies in the emphasis of their work. The major responsibilities of these technologists are in the area of diagnostic testing, while the respiratory therapist is more deeply involved in therapeutic (treatment) aspects of pulmonary technology. Some technologists work in both the cardiac and pulmonary areas. They, as you might suspect, are professionally known as cardiopulmonary technologists.

These job titles commonly used today are in a state of flux. Efforts are under way on the part of physicians and technologists working in the cardiac field to adopt "cardiovascular technologist" as the recognized official occupational title for technologists who have been trained in both non-invasive and invasive cardiac procedures. Although they are trained in both procedures, technologists may function exclusively in one or in both. In recent years, the title "cardiopulmonary technologist" has been used for professionals who have even broader knowledge. In addition to knowing invasive and non-invasive cardiovascular procedures, the cardiopulmonary technologist has expertise in the pulmonary area.

It probably will take several years before these job titles gain wide acceptance.

In the meanwhile, cardiopulmonary specialists continue to perform a vital role in health care, regardless of what's in the name.

RESPONSIBILITIES

Thus far you have met the cardiopulmonary specialist in name only. On the job he or she is involved in a wide range of procedures, working with the physician to obtain the necessary diagnostic information or to give treatment. One may work in the cardiopulmonary laboratory or at the patient's bedside in the intensive care or regular patient unit. The professional responsibilities vary a great deal, depending on the employer for whom the specialist works and the specific procedures which he is required to perform. But no matter what the procedures, the technologist's basic responsibilities lie with the patient, the machine, and the test or treatment results.

There is no categorizing the patients with whom the technologist works, short of saying that they have (or are suspected of having) lung or heart problems, or both. Some are pediatric patients, born with congenital (meaning at birth) defects which rob them of their cardiopulmonary function. Others are victims of progressive arteriosclerotic heart disease, commonly known as hardening of the arteries. (This disease narrows their blood vessels, thereby placing an increasing strain upon the heart.) Victims of emphysema, asthma, or other respiratory problems are also among the patients seen in the pulmonary laboratory. Each patient's particular condition dictates which test(s) their physican will order. But not all patients are ill. Many undergo routine evaluations to assess the basic functioning of both these organ systems.

During examinations, the technologist must carefully monitor both the patient and the machine. Patient observation is particularly important. Many patients may be ill or in poor physical condition. The examination, though carefully controlled, may make unusual demands upon the body, the results of which cannot be predicted. This could range from simple fatigue, which necessitates halting the procedure, to a more serious problem, such as a heart attack or respiratory failure, which would require immediate medical attention. With invasive procedures, particularly when a dye or other substance is injected into the body, results can be unpredictable. Though 99 out of 100 patients will have no reaction, there is always that 1% possibility. Clearly, the technologist must be vigilant when working with patients.

The machine must first be set up and then constantly monitored. Improper use of the equipment or machine malfunction may give false information. This could mislead the physician into making the wrong diagnosis. Since the equipment is electrically operated, the technologist must be alert to electrical safety—not only for the patient, but for himself.

Finally, the test (or treatment) results must be organized and presented to the physician so that he or she can quickly review the information and reach a conclusion. In the case of the EKG reading, this may consist of nothing more than removing the paper upon which the tracings were recorded from the EKG machine, and then cutting, editing, and mounting the tracings for the physician's use. In a pulmonary study, for example, it may involve first calculating carbon dioxide or oxygen levels present, plotting the results on a graph, and then supplementing the examination report with observation notes. Records which the technologist keeps are extremely important. The results of patients' tests may be kept for years; therefore, they must be well organized, contain all necessary identifying information, and be carefully filed and stored so that they will be available for immediate use.

In addition to recordkeeping, there are frequently other administrative duties. Equipment supplies must be ordered, patients must be scheduled, and work must be organized. Depending on the technologist's level of responsibility within the department, more or less of these duties will be required. The technologist's duties may also vary from employer to employer.

But the best way to really understand what cardiopulmonary technology is all about is to spend a few hours in a cardiac and then in a pulmonary laboratory. Some hospitals today have combined these diagnostic services into a single cardiopulmonary laboratory staffed by technologists fully equipped and trained in both areas.

INSIDE THE HOSPITAL

It is not quite 9:00 A.M. You have to hurry. Before your first patient arrives, everything in the laboratory must be double-checked and in order for the day's procedures. Emergency drugs and oxygen are ready and on hand in case they will be needed. The patient charts have been pulled. Your equipment has been checked and is in good working order. You are now ready for Mr. Elverson, your first patient. He is typical of many of your patients: middle-aged, slightly overweight, and no longer very physically active. Lately, he has been bothered by mild chest pains after moderate physical labor. Gas pains, he insists, but his family physician has referred him to your laboratory for evaluation. Dr. Stempien, the cardiologist, has already reviewed his physician's referral slip and has okayed the basic evaluation for this patient. Later, after your tests have been completed and he has examined Mr. Elverson himself, Dr. Stempien will review the entire case again before reaching any conclusions.

Mr. Elverson is nervously waiting outside. You introduce yourself and usher him into the examination room. You urge him to relax. There will be nothing mysterious about today's procedures, you explain. First you will be taking a simple EKG while he is at rest. Then he will undergo a cardiac stress test, which will test his heart during physical activity. Before you begin the actual examination, you take a simple patient history which emphasizes factors related to his heart. You are interested not only in his own history, but in whether or not any immediate family members may have had cardiac problems. This will help Dr. Stempien determine whether there may be a genetic reason for any ailment he may uncover.

You question him about past illnesses and his personal habits. Does he smoke or drink? If so, how much each day? Does he exercise regularly? What kind of stress does he experience during his regular working day? Does he take any medications? All this information helps develop a cardiac profile of your patient.

You show him to the changing room, and instruct him to remove his shirt. During the EKG he will be resting on an examination table. Contrary to what most people think, the EKG does not record the muscular action of his heart; instead, it records the heart's electrical action. You now prepare Mr. Elverson for the examination. You attach electrodes on his chest, arms, and legs, and then you test your machine to make sure it is not recording any outside stimulus such as the tremors of his muscles or electrical vibrations from other nearby equipment. "What do I do now?" he asks. "You do nothing," you reply. All he has to do during this exam is simply lie there. "Your work will come next, during the stress test." Soon the examination is over and you remove the electrodes from Mr. Elverson. "That was fast," he says. "The stress test will take a little longer," you explain. You carefully notate the EKG record and prepare him for the next test. Again, electrodes will be used, but this time extra ones will be attached. In addition to monitoring his heart during activity, a special electrode will be recording his blood pressure throughout the examination. You attach the electrodes and calibrate your equipment. You notice one of the tracings is a little abnormal, so you double-check the electrode. Sure enough, you are picking up some of his muscle action, and you move the electrode slightly to compensate. The artifact disappears. Now you are ready to begin. You ask Mr. Elverson to step on the treadmill. You explain that once the treadmill is moving he should walk at a normal pace. "And then you want me to jog?" he asks. "No," you explain, "you will be walking throughout the entire exam." "Just walking?" he questions. "Yes, that's right. But you will see, even without jogging, your heart will do a great deal of work." Instead of the treadmill going faster, you explain, the angle of the treadmill will be elevated slowly. "Sort of like walking uphill?" he asks. "That's it exactly." You caution him not to hold on to the handrails. If he needs to use them for balance, he may place only a finger or two on them. His heart must do all the work, unassisted. The examination begins.

The treadmill starts moving slowly at the leisurely pace of window shopping. You caution him to let you know when he begins to experience any pain. During the stress test you will be monitoring him carefully. Some patients try to outperform their bodies and refuse to "give in," though they may be experiencing pain. As soon as you observe this behavior you must call the examination to a halt before the patient reaches a critical point. Other patients react oppositely, trying to call the examination "quits" before their heart has really reached its maximum work capacity. You must encourage these patients to work harder. Once Mr. Elverson is accustomed to the treadmill, you slowly begin elevating its angle. You start first with a 5% incline. The heart rate changes slightly. You continue for several minutes and then increase the grade again. Now he is walking at a 10% incline. "How are you feeling? you ask. "Fine," he replies. "No problem." After several minutes you increase the grade slightly again. Now you can see a change in your patient. His heart is having to work much harder and he is beginning to tire. Beads of perspiration are forming on his forehead. "Are you experiencing any pain yet?" you ask. "No," he says, "I am fine." You continue to watch his heart action and blood pressure recordings carefully. He may be one of those patients who feels he has to prove something. Mr. Elverson calls out. He says he is starting to feel those old pains again. "I guess this time I can't say it is gas." Your readings indicate that his heart is working very hard now and without regularity. It is time to stop. You tell Mr. Elverson that you are turning off the machine now. "But," he says, "the pains aren't that bad. I can still . . ." You cut him off quickly. "We are stopping." You hand him some Kleenex so he can mop his brow. You slowly remove each of the electrodes. "How did I do?" "Just fine," you tell him. "You can put your shirt on now." "That's it?" he asks. "That's it. At least with me, at any rate." You tell him that he will soon be seeing Dr. Stempien.

While Mr. Elverson is in the changing room, you are organizing his records and the results of your examination for Dr. Stempien's review. When Mr. Elverson returns, he eyes his EKG with interest. You point out to him the spot where his heart began working harder. He can see himself the marked difference between his resting and working EKG. You shake hands and thank him for his cooperation.

You now get ready for your next patient. This, again, is a stress test, but your patient, Mrs. Frost, is here for a special evaluation. This woman suffered a heart attack just three months ago and is now in the reconditioning stage, gradually returning to normal activities and exercise. This stress testing will help evaluate how well her heart is recovering and help Dr. Stempien plan her reconditioning program. You already have a history for this patient, but you question her about her recent activities and whether or not she has experienced any chest pains or unusual experiences. You then prepare the patient and the equipment for the examination. The examination goes well. Her heart is recovering nicely. Her reaction to the test was similar to that of many other heart attack patients: Instead of being nervous about the examination, afraid it might bring on another attack, she felt secure knowing that you and Dr. Stempien were there in case anything should happen. Also, she can now see on paper the real progress she has made in just twelve weeks.

You receive a call from the pediatric unit. A physician needs a special phonocardiograph on a four-month-old patient. The baby was born with a defect in the valves of the heart, and this phonocardiograph examination will help the physician to evaluate the extent of the problem. The phonocardiograph is nothing more than an electronic stethoscope which picks up the sound of the heart valves, amplifies it, and then displays it in graph form. While it does not provide any more information than a conventional stethoscope, it is useful because it provides the physican with a permanent record of the baby's heartbeat which can be analyzed and discussed with other physicians.

Upon returning to the lab you are greeted by Mr. Newman, who has returned his holter monitoring tape. This is a special 24-hour electrocardiogram reading. Yesterday, when he came into the cardiac lab, you attached the special holter monitoring unit to his body, which he wore for a full 24-hour period. The entire unit weighed just a few pounds and was no heavier than carrying around a light briefcase. During that 24-hour period, while the holter monitor did its work, your patient had to do work too. He had to keep a special diary in which he noted any time he experienced chest pains or other problems. He carefully noted the time, what he was doing specifically, and how he felt. Though his tape ran for 24 hours, each minute was condensed, so that his 24-hour tape will take you only an hour and a half to play back. You will view it on a special oscilloscope screen and notate the record when you notice areas of particular interest or significance. This will then be matched against Mr. Newman's diary, thereby saving Dr. Stempien time and giving him a more comprehensive picture of this patient's particular problem. Mr. Newman himself explains that he learned a great deal from keeping the diary. Much of the chest pain he experienced was not the result of physical exercise, but the result of stress he experienced on his job.

You break for lunch now. You are meeting Ms. Rockwell, a technologist who works in a cardiac catheterization lab. This procedure with which she works daily is highly specialized. It helps to diagnose accurately and objectively the extent of heart disease prior to surgery. She assists the physician as he inserts a catheter (a tube) of radio-opaque nylon, just two millimeters in diameter, into a vein in the patient's right arm. Once a catheter is inserted, the physician then injects heparin, a drug, immediately into the bloodstream to prevent blood clotting. The catheter is filled with saline (salt) to prevent air from entering the blood. The physician slowly pushes the catheter through the vein until it reaches the superior vena cava, one of the large veins that drain directly into the heart. During this time the progress of the catheter is being observed on the fluoroscope. Then, depending on the readings the physician wishes to make, the catheter can be pushed into the right side of the heart to record blood pressure. Also, the oxygen level can be determined by withdrawing a blood sample directly from the catheter. Special dyes can also be injected through the catheter into the heart and a series of rapid or still X-ray pictures taken. During this procedure Ms. Rockwell performs many activities to assist the physician. She positions and keeps the patient immobile if necessary, prepares the syringes containing the dye, and takes and analyzes the blood samples from the catheter as it passes through various areas of the heart. She may also, at the physician's request, take the radiographic study.

Because catheterization is considered a surgical procedure, the catheterization lab in which the procedure takes place resembles a mini operating room. Everything must be done under completely sterile conditions. As you might well imagine, the procedure is a tricky one and requires great skill on the part of the physician.

After lunch you are off to the pulmonary laboratory. As yet your hospital has not combined this laboratory with the cardiac lab, but may do so in the near future. Heart and lung function are closely related, and many of your patients who are studied in one lab must also be examined in the other.

Judy Jacksina, a spritely teenager, is your first patient for the afternoon. She suffers from frequent asthma attacks, which have been getting worse. You will be doing a spirometry test to measure her breathing capacity and the volume of her lungs. You explain the procedure and ask her to put the mouthpiece in place. You instruct her to breathe normally through the spirometer until she is accustomed to the unusual sensation. "How are you doing?" you ask. She smiles with the mouthpiece still in place. "Okay," you explain, "now we will try the nose clips." You put the nose clips on and instruct her to just keep breathing normally. You notice a strange look on her face and ask her if everything is all right. She nods in assent. You give her hand a little squeeze and tell her to relax. You are ready now to take the actual lung measurement. You ask her to breathe as deeply as she can while you measure the volume and the flow rate. This is all done with special equipment which automatically records the results. Some equipment is computerized; however, this model is not, so after you have obtained the measurements you must translate this data into the diagnostic information the physician needs. While Judy is breathing into the equipment, you watch her carefully. You must be sure that there are no leaks from her mouth or nose which would invalidate the test results. Soon the examination is over and you can remove the clamps and mouthpiece. Judy smiles. It feels good to breathe naturally again.

Dr. Bush enters and asks you to report to the intensive care unit. He would like you to evaluate the pulmonary function of a critically ill patient whose breathing is assisted by a ventilator. No machine, no matter how expertly designed, can ever completely take over for the human body's own organs. You will be testing how well this ventilator is supporting the patient's oxygen needs.

You head immediately for the intensive care unit. As soon as you arrive you check in with the nurse on duty. Mr. Fitzsimons, as head nurse, is responsible for everything that goes on in the intensive care unit. Other health professionals entering the I.C.U. must clear through him first. He pulls the patient's chart for you to quickly review and then shows you to the patient's room. You now begin your procedure. The patient will remain on the ventilator all the time you do your work. You first collect an air sample from the air which the patient has just exhaled, by opening the expiratory portion of the ventilator. This air is collected in a special bag which you have brought with you. This will be needed for gas analysis. Meanwhile Ms. Mitchell, another technologist, is noting the patient's age, height, and weight from his record, which you will need for computational purposes later. Then, together, you draw an arterial blood sample. She holds the arm immobile while you carefully take the blood. Taking an arterial sample requires great care because the blood is under tremendous pressure. A sudden movement on the

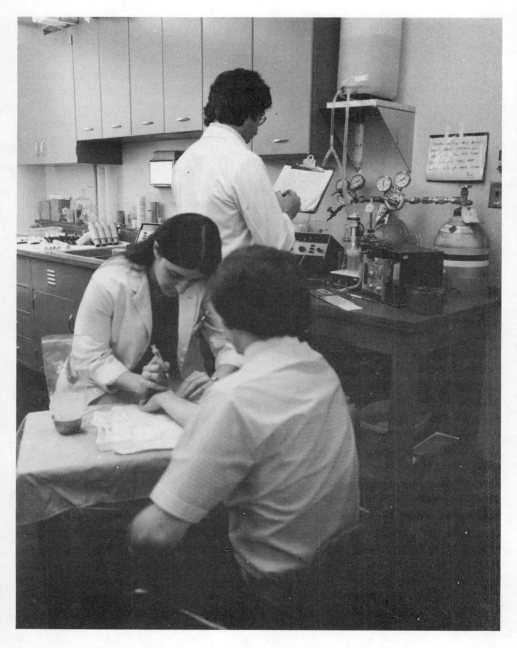

The analysis of arterial blood gases enables technologists to evaluate cardiopulmonary function. Courtesy of Ohio State University.

patient's part could be damaging. You remove the blood sample, cap it, and place it in a container of crushed ice and water. Then you and Ms. Mitchell return to the cardiopulmonary laboratory with your two samples. You carefully calibrate your analyzers, making sure, before you run your tests, that they are in top working order. You will be recording the pH level, the PO_2 and the PCO_2 levels—the oxygen and carbon dioxide levels which are recorded under pressure—of the patient's blood. You are ready now for the actual analysis. You withdraw a 15-millimeter sample of the expired air in the collection bag, and slowly inject it through one of the analyzers. The machine then measures the partial pressures of both oxygen and carbon dioxide in the expired air sample. The remaining volume of air in the bag is then measured, using a dry gas meter. You must then adjust your figure for the number of millimeters which were already removed and for the atmospheric pressure and the room temperature. Meanwhile, Ms. Mitchell is analyzing the blood sample. When you both have finished the many and varied calculations, the physician will have a good picture of the patient's respiration at the most basic cellular level. Your data analysis will tell the physician whether the ventilator must be adjusted or if the therapy for this patient must be changed.

Because blood gas analyses give the physician so much information on pulmonary function, this test is one that you perform frequently. In fact, your next procedure will again involve a blood gas analysis. However, this time the test will take you to the preemie unit, where you will be obtaining a blood sample from a baby born just days ago, but weeks too soon. Before heading to the preemie unit, you make sure that you have all your sterile supplies—the syringe, antiseptic solution, sterile needles, cotton, and a tube already marked for your young patient's blood sample.

You again check in with the nurse in charge upon arrival. Your littlest patient has been struggling for life these last few days. His lungs are not yet fully capable of doing the work required, so they must be assisted. As with the ventilated patient, these blood gas analyses again will tell the physician how well this most basic human need is being met. On such a tiny baby it would be impossible to draw the blood from an arm or a leg. Instead, the sample will be taken from his umbilical cord, which is still partially intact. With great skill and accuracy you enter the needle into the umbilicus and withdraw the needed sample. Minutes later you are back at your workbench in the laboratory, analyzing the function of his tiny lungs. The readings look good. Chances are the little guy will make it.

The rest of the afternoon passes uneventfully. You do two more blood gas analyses, some pulmonary exercise stress testing, and a pre-operative test for lung function. Throughout the afternoon you are constantly busy, working with patients, making various calculations, and plotting and graphing results for the physicians. Finally, before the day is over, you do a simple maintenance check on the machines and recalibrate them for tomorrow's activities. Then it is time to go home. You think about tomorrow and wonder what will it bring.

What will *your* tomorrow bring? Could it possibly hold a career working in one or both of these vital areas?

PERSONAL QUALIFICATIONS AND WORKING CONDITIONS

Good observation, accuracy, thoroughness, and an eye for detail are important qualities for persons working in the cardiopulmonary field. These skills are necessary in order to perform the many and varied diagnostic tests or treatment procedures. Organizational ability is important as well, not only for organizing test results and patient information, but for carrying out various administrative and departmental duties, such as scheduling patients and ordering equipment and supplies. Because technologists work closely with people, whether they be patients, patients' families, or physicians, good communication skills are an important asset. Because of the close human contact, sensitivity and genuine interest in people are important. Technologists, in performing many tests, must be able to encourage the patient and bring out the best performance possible. This requires a special combination of tact, patience, and psychology.

Technologists, whether they are working in the cardiology or pulmonary area or a combination of both, generally work a 40-hour week. In large hospitals, evening and weekend work on a rotating basis may be required. In general, there are no unusual physical demands required for persons working in cardiopulmonary technology. Some lifting or positioning of patients may be required, but usually this is kept to a minimum.

PREPARING FOR TRAINING

Because the field of cardiopulmonary technology is so broad, a good general preparation in science and math is recommended. Clearly, the more science and math you study during high school or college, the better will be your foundation upon which later training can build. The stronger the foundation, the more prepared the student will be to move into the more complex areas within the technology. Since this job involves working closely with people, courses which will improve communication skills, such as English, reading, and writing, as well as those which deal with one's understanding of people, such as psychology and sociology, are also helpful.

PROFESSIONAL TRAINING

Traditionally, most persons working in cardiopulmonary technology, with the exception of those in respiratory therapy, have been trained on the job (OJT). Some formal preparation in cardiopulmonary technology is available through military training programs. Though on-the-job training is still offered in some health facilities, formal education programs are now available and are strongly recommended because they offer the students the greatest opportunities for eventual career advancement. In those places where on-the-job training is still being conducted, requirements for a trainee's position will be determined by each employer.

In general, to perform non-invasive cardiac testing requires, at minimum, a high school education. Some college, with an emphasis on science and/or related work experience, is usually required to qualify for on-the-job training in invasive cardiac testing. The length of training also varies. Three to six months of on-the-job training is generally required to become proficient in one non-invasive test such as the EKG. To gain competency in additional tests would require more OJT. Invasive procedures would require still more extensive training, usually six to twelve months. Training in both non-invasive and invasive areas would cover the fundamentals of equipment operation and maintenance, basic heart and chest anatomy, electrical safety, and emergency first aid procedures, including cardiopulmonary resuscitation. This classroom work would be combined with *closely* supervised experience with patients.

Formal education programs leading to a certificate or an associate degree in cardiology technology are offered by hospitals, community colleges, universities, and technical institutes. Some of these programs involve only non-invasive techniques, while others combine study in both invasive and non-invasive procedures, thereby producing a graduate well equipped to perform in the most general areas of the hospital cardiology laboratory. The American Cardiology Technologists Association (ACTA) currently sponsors an accreditation program in this particular field.

A program which is accredited by ACTA will cover basic medical terminology, English, math, anatomy and physiology, and elementary physics. The specialized curriculum will cover basic electrocardiography and specialized techniques such as vectorcardiography and phonocardiography, stress testing, or holter monitoring. A basic orientation to echocardiography is also required. In addition, the student must receive a minimum of 480 hours of clinical experience. The length of training in cardiology or cardiopulmonary technology varies, but generally these requirements cannot be met in less than a one- to two-year program, in addition to specific entrance prerequisites.

Programs specifically designed to prepare students to function in both cardiac and pulmonary areas are accredited by the National Society for Cardiopulmonary Technology. In addition to certificate and associate degree programs, a few universities offer a four-year bachelor's degree. Because these programs must cover both the cardiac, invasive and non-invasive, and the pulmonary fields, they are intensive. Programs include coursework in the basic sciences such as physics, math, chemistry, anatomy, and physiology. The specialized curriculum covers cardiovascular pharmacology, medical electronics, basic medical instrumentation, fundamentals of pulmonary and cardiovascular physiology, and the application of technology to these areas. In addition, according to the Society guidelines, intensive clinical experience is required—at least 1,000 hours.

Admission requirements for all programs vary tremendously. Some programs admit students directly from high school. Others require one to two years of college work, with an emphasis on the basic sciences, before admission.

In order to be considered for admission, a student must complete an application form; a personal interview may be required, as well as special admissions tests. Because there are so few programs in this area, schools can be selective in their admissions process. Costs vary with the program itself. Generally, little tuition is charged by hospital programs and community colleges, while university programs must charge tuition rates comparable to other programs.

Because programs are so individual, it is best to start investigating various programs as early as possible so that you can compare curriculums and clinical experience that each program offers. In general, programs offering education and training in a wide variety of techniques, coupled with extensive clinical preparation, will offer the greatest job opportunities both immediately following graduation and in the future.

PROFESSIONAL CREDENTIALS

At the present time there is no licensure required for persons working in the cardiopulmonary field. The National Society for Cardiopulmonary Technology certifies, by examination, technologists working in this field. The certification is actually a two-step process. The first step is the completion of a general examination covering cardiopulmonary, anatomy, physiology, pathology and medical electronics, and basic methods in cardiopulmonary technology, both invasive and non-invasive techniques. After completing this general examination, technologists are eligible to sit for a more intensive registry examination, either in cardiopulmonary technology or its specialized areas, cardiovascular technology or pulmonary technology. Upon successful completion of this examination, technologists may use the designation R-CPT, registered cardiopulmonary technologist; R-CVT, cardiovascular technologist; or R-PuT, registered pulmonary technologist.

The American Cardiology Technologists Association (ACTA) also offers a certification program for technologists working specifically in the cardiology area. After completing the ACTA examination, technologists are designated RCT, registered cardiology technologists.

Certification is not required for employment. However, it does assure employers that technologists who hold these designations are competent in their field. In many instances higher salaries are paid to technologists who hold certification. In addition to salary increases, opportunities for advancement within the field generally are more available to certified technologists.

JOB OPPORTUNITIES

Cardiovascular disease is our number-one killer, and, as a result of smoking and air pollution, pulmonary disease is on the rise.

The increasing reliance on cardiac and pulmonary tests to diagnose heart, lung, and circulatory disease makes the employment outlook in this field promising. Many institutions which have not been practicing this technology in the past are now instituting cardiopulmonary laboratories, creating a need for educated and experienced technologists. Presently there is a shortage of trained, qualified personnel who can perform the highly specialized duties of a cardiopulmonary technologist. Opportunities for technologists who perform only one particular cardiac non-invasive test are limited without higher education. Though hospitals, clinics, and private physicians' offices have traditionally been the major employers of those working in cardiopulmonary technology, opportunities are expanding to include home care facilities, environmentally related institutions, industrial facilities, and even mobile testing units.

Starting salaries vary tremendously according to the scope of the technologist's responsibilities. Depending on local salaries, a starting "EKG technician" may earn between $7,000 and $9,500 per year, while a technologist trained in both invasive and non-invasive cardiology techniques will begin about $3,000 higher, as will the cardiopulmonary technologist.

THE PIONEER SPIRIT

If a field is still brand new and even the job titles aren't definite yet, should you get involved? "In a word, yes," said one technologist. "I'm here on the inside of what is going to be one of the most important diagnostic areas yet. Jobs in my field are increasing with the greater emphasis on prevention—even many employers are sending their personnel for evaluations. As I see it, I'm a pioneer learning and growing with the field. As for the job titles, that doesn't bother me; what counts is that I have a career that's needed in health care today."

For additional information on careers and professional credentials write:

American Cardiology Technologists Association
1 Bank Street
Gaithersburg, MD 20760

National Society for Cardiopulmonary Technology
1 Bank Street
Gaithersburg, MD 20760

CHAPTER VIII

Harnessing Human Electricity

Whether you realize it or not, your brain is an extremely complex organ containing almost ten billion nerve cells. It is your body's master control organ that regulates most of your body functions. Without proper brain function, more than just your ability to think is impaired. Your ability to see, touch, talk, and coordinate your body are all affected. Vital body functions such as temperature, heart rate, and breathing are affected as well. Your blood pressure, sleep and waking cycles, appetite, thirst, hormonal cycles, and emotional behavior are but a few of the many other areas for which your brain acts as the vital control mechanism. Even as you read these pages now, your brain is reacting to the written messages which it receives.

How does your brain signal the rest of the body? The precise process is not completely understood, but we know that the brain gives off electrical impulses, impulses so small that they must be measured in millionths of a volt. Yet despite their microvoltage these signals can be picked up, amplified, and recorded by a special machine—the electroencephalograph, more commonly called the EEG machine.

The study of the brain's electrical wave patterns in both normal and abnormal patients is the basis of the medical science known as electroencephalography. Just as in the other branches of medical science, in electroencephalography the physician does not work alone but is assisted by the allied health specialists, the EEG technician and technologist.

THE EEG IN MEDICINE TODAY

As a medical tool, the EEG is a diagnostic key which helps to confirm a variety of brain disorders—epilepsy, brain tumors, stroke, certain infections. With some disorders, such as epilepsy, the EEG is *the* medical test which determines the diagnosis, while in other brain problems the EEG makes a valuable addition to medical information. When used in cooperation with other tests, the EEG gives the physician a more complete picture of what is happening to the patient.

Any problem which may be linked to the brain is a potential case for the EEG specialist. For example, the EEG may be used to determine if there is a physical reason for a patient's erratic emotional behavior or a child's learning difficulties.

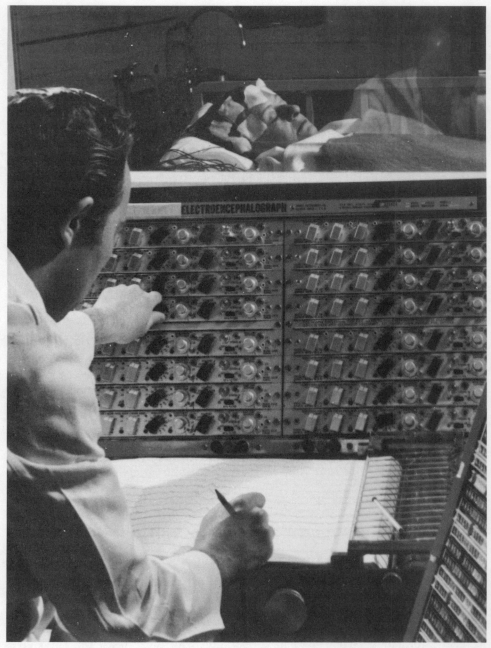

EEG technologist conducts an examination. Courtesy of National Institutes of Health.

But the EEG is not only used to diagnose brain disorders. It can also assist in diagnosing other problems, such as those related to human metabolism, kidney, or liver disorders. Since the advent of organ transplants, the Living Will, and the Right to Die With Dignity movement, another use of the EEG has become well publicized. It is used to determine death. The confirmation of whether a patient is alive or dead no longer depends on the mere presence or absence of a heartbeat. In medical circles "brain death," as established via the EEG, has become the chief, though sometimes still controversial, criterion.

But whether the EEG is used to determine disability, disease, or brain death, EEG specialists are the allied health professionals who actually perform the examinations. Once completed, their test results are turned over to the echoencephalographer. This is a physician, often a neurologist or neurosurgeon, who is specially trained to interpret the EEG examination.

THE EEG SPECIALIST AND THE PATIENT

There is no categorizing the patients whom the EEG specialist meets. Problems related to brain activity may strike at any age.

Specialists work with a wide range of patients, from preemie babies, whose gestational age can be determined by the maturity of their brain wave patterns, to elderly stroke victims. The mental and physical condition of their patients varies too. Some may be alert and without apparent problems, while others may be in severe pain or emotional distress, semi-conscious, or in a comatose state. Each patient is unique; each examination presents a new and different challenge to the specialist.

In order to perform an EEG examination, the specialist must work closely with the patient. This interaction begins even before the exam itself. As soon as the specialist and patient meet, the stage is being set for the examination which will follow.

Patient relaxation is important for a good examination. The EEG machine is so sensitive that even the blink of an eye will be recorded on the EEG tracings. Tension, psychological stress, and other factors can be reflected in the brain wave tracings, thereby decreasing the accuracy of the exam.

The skilled EEG specialist immediately makes the patient feel as much at ease as possible, and then carefully explains the examination procedure. The patient dialogue doesn't end here. Another key element in a good exam is the patient's clinical history. If the specialist is lucky, the patient's history will be available for review before the examination begins. However, in many cases it has not been sent to the EEG lab in advance. The only way the specialist can obtain it is by asking the patient directly.

Once the patient has been prepared and the examination begins, an average EEG takes about 45 minutes to complete. During that time the specialist's attention is concentrated on the patient, the machine, and the EEG recordings. Mechanical malfunctions which could invalidate the test results must be caught. More importantly, the specialist must closely observe the patient's behavior, not only for signs of an emergency, such as an impending seizure, but so that the specialist can later correlate the patient's clinical condition (drowsiness, fully awake, etc.) with the appropriate EEG tracings.

Not all work with patients takes place inside the EEG department. Some special patient studies take the specialist to the emergency room, the operating room, the intensive care unit, or regular patient floors. Often these special studies require the EEG specialist to modify or adapt their standard techniques.

Wherever specialists work, the examination itself is their primary responsibility, but it is by no means their only one.

ADDITIONAL RESPONSIBILITIES

To the unskilled eye, an EEG recording looks like a series of wiggly pen lines on paper, almost like a child's scribbling.

Translating or "interpreting" the EEG results so that they have medical meaning requires tremendous skill and experience. Even a very subtle change in electrical wave activity can be important. EEG interpretation is a role reserved for physicians only. However, the EEG specialist plays an important part in helping to organize the test data.

Throughout the exam, EEG tracings are being recorded on paper. This results in a volume of clinical data. To help the physician quickly sift through the information, the specialist not only observes the patient and machine during the exam, but takes clinical notes. Some notes may indicate a particular activity the patient was asked to perform; others may indicate the patient's level of consciousness during a specific portion of the exam. The specialist, as the on-the-spot observer, may also alert the doctor to any part of the examination which may be unusual or of possible clinical significance. Depending on the policy in some institutions, EEG specialists also summarize or "abstract" their clinical impressions of the examinations as an additional aid to the physician.

Like any other allied health professional who works with special biomedical equipment, the EEG specialist must know machine basics: whether the instrument is working properly, whether it is properly calibrated, and, if a minor problem exists—such as a tube blowout—how to correct it. More serious problems are usually handled by a biomedical equipment technician or a staff electrical engineer.

In some health facilities, the EEG specialist may also be involved with such basic department operations as appointment scheduling, ordering supplies, and laboratory recordkeeping.

TECHNOLOGIST VS. TECHNICIAN

Before going any deeper into the EEG field, you should understand the differences between the technologist and the technician. Both are fully qualified to perform the EEG examination. As with most allied health professions which recognize a "technician" and a "technologist" level, the technologist has received more extensive training.

This gives the EEG technologist greater opportunities to eventually tackle more extensive job responsibilities. These might include department supervision, teaching, and administration. Other areas where the technologist's education may lead are working with physicians on EEG and brain research or handling more complicated patient examinations. Complicated cases often require the specialist to modify standard EEG techniques to the patient's specific problems. It is also the technologist who is usually called upon to write a descriptive report of the clinical EEG findings.

Those who choose EEG as a lifetime career and enter the field via the technician's route should consider this level just the first step—the bottom step of a two-rung ladder. Most technicians usually advance to the technologist level through additional training and/or job experience.

ON THE JOB

If you were to choose EEG as a career, what would your workday be like? Join these technologists on the job and see for yourself.

Your weekly scheduled in-service training program is about to begin. The staff—physicians, EEG technologists, and technicians—have already assembled in the conference room. Patients will be seen later in the day. This time is devoted to reviewing interesting patient cases and to discussing new technological developments. This is one part of your job which you find particularly interesting. It gives you an opportunity to learn more about your chosen field.

You listen intently as the various patient records are read and discussed by the physicians. You have a great interest in the case which is currently being discussed—the case of Frank Brady, one of your patients. The neurologist is using this case to illustrate how the EEG can be useful in making a diagnosis of hepatitis. He calls upon you to describe the patient's clinical condition and the wave patterns which were recorded. Later, after all the clinical cases have been discussed, there is a demonstration of some new equipment by a manufacturer's representative. When the demonstration and question-and-answer period are over, the in-service training session ends. You hurry off to your first patient.

Mrs. McKerrow is waiting inside the examination room. She seems quite nervous and constantly fidgets in her seat. You already see that unless you can get her to relax, this examination will be difficult. You smile, introduce yourself, and ask her how she feels today. "Good," she replies cautiously.

You review her chart. It indicates her family physician has referred her to the EEG lab for "headaches." Almost no other information, except identification, has been included in the requisition slip.

You carefully explain the EEG examination procedure and assure her that it is absolutely painless. You also tell her that it *cannot* "read" her thoughts. It doesn't act as a lie detector either. She seems to relax a bit now.

You begin to take a brief clinical history, questioning her about her headaches. "When did your headaches start?" you ask. "Did they occur at a particular time of day? Where are they located? Do they recur under periods of stress? While you are having a headache are you bothered by lights? Or do you feel nauseated? Do you feel nauseated at a particular time of the day—for example, when you get up?"

You ask these questions to see if there is a pattern to her headaches, one which may indicate migraine headaches or headaches caused by a possible tumor. For example, if the headaches and nausea are experienced together, upon rising, this could be a sign of a tumor. Her answers point strongly toward a classic migraine pattern.

Now that you have the clinical information that you need, you prepare Mrs. McKerrow for the examination. Before you begin applying the electrodes that will pick up the brain's wave patterns, you carefully clean the scalp area where each electrode will be attached. This helps to remove fats, oils, and dead skin—all substances which would interfere with electrical conducting. You measure her head and then start to apply the electrodes. You add a jelly between the electrode and the scalp. This acts as a conducting aid.

Occasionally you use special needle electrodes. Today, however, you are working with small silver disks, which will be attached directly to the patient's scalp and connected to the EEG machine by wires and plug, almost like a telephone switchboard. To hold the electrodes in place you will use a special substance called collodion, which resembles a heavy sticky hairspray. Adhesive caps, clay, or paraffin may also be used to hold the electrodes in place. Sometimes, too, electrodes are mounted in a special headband which can be strapped to the patient's skull.

You start arranging the electrodes in a predetermined pattern. Your lab uses the international 10-20 system of electrode placement. When the last electrode is in place, you ask Mrs. McKerrow to recline on the couch. "Just close your eyes and relax," you urge her. Meanwhile you have turned on the EEG machine and are carefully checking to see that it is correctly calibrated, the recording pens are in place, and the entire machine is working properly. You notice a strange signal and check the machine to determine the cause of the artifact. You adjust the dials for frequency and amplitude, but the signal remains. It disappears, however, when you slightly reposition one of Mrs. McKerrow's electrodes, which had been resting on an artery in the scalp. Just a few millimeters is enough to make a difference.

Now the examination officially begins. You again ask Mrs. McKerrow to close her eyes and relax. Try concentrating on something pleasant, you suggest. Soon her brain wave patterns change and the EEG begins to pick up her "alpha waves." She opens her eyes and blinks and the waves suddenly disappear. The EEG machine is so sensitive that eye blinks, a mouth opening or closing, or swallowing can be detected. You notate the EEG records and gently remind her to keep her eyes closed and to move as little as possible. The alpha waves soon appear again.

Throughout the examination you monitor your patient, the machine, and the EEG recording. Monitoring the recording itself takes a lot of skill and practice. On this particular test you are using eight channels. (Some machines record up to eighteen.) This means that the EEG pens are producing eight separate tracings and wave patterns. The patterns correspond to various electrode pairs on the patient's skull. Different electrode pair combinations are recorded at different times during the exam. Each particular sequence of eight is a separate "montage."

While your patient is relaxed, you are very, very busy. You continue taking notes. At one point you notice that Mrs. McKerrow's brain waves are changing. You observe your patient. Sure enough, she is starting to fall asleep. You rouse her gently; she must be alert during the examination. The rest of the examination proceeds uneventfully. Afterwards, you remove the electrodes and the collodion from the patient's scalp. By now Mrs. McKerrow and you are chatting like old friends. There is no sign of the anxious woman who first greeted you. As she leaves, you remind her to check with her doctor in a few days for the test results.

Your next patient, Lauren Rogers, looks like a healthy youngster about seven years old. Yet, despite her appearance, her patient chart indicates a history of erratic behavior and possible seizures. Diagnosis, probable epilepsy.

You question her mother about her behavior, and ask when she last had a "seizure." This information is particularly important. If the seizure was recent, her brain wave patterns may be changed temporarily. You have to alter your technique to ascertain whether Lauren's pattern indicates epilepsy, a disorder whose cause is still unknown, or may be caused by another condition, perhaps a structural problem in the brain.

You explain the entire EEG procedure to Lauren's mother and, in a few simple steps, to Lauren. You then start preparing your young patient for the examination. Instead of being frightened by the exam and requiring some sedation, as many children do, she is excited and talks nonstop about her pets, schoolwork, and two older sisters, Kirsten and Megan. After you have applied the last electrode, you pull out a small mirror from a desk drawer and hand it to her. She gazes at herself admiringly in the mirror and exclaims, "I'm a Indian chief." You both laugh.

You then turn on the machine and carefully check its functioning. All the time she is watching you with great curiosity. You explain what you are doing and what the machine is picking up. You promise her a surprise at the end of the examination if she will try hard to follow your instructions. It is a deal! You explain that she must close her eyes and keep as still as a mouse. No talking or moving, you explain. Just play possum. Her mother sits nearby, quietly watching.

The EEG pens begin recording her brain wave pattern. They are lively and fast— totally different from an adult's brain waves, yet for a child completely normal. The pattern continues for a short time and then begins to change. You can tell by the pattern that a seizure is approaching. Because all her seizures have been very mild in the past and have not required any emergency medical attention, you do not call the doctor now. Instead you observe her behavior even more closely and take very careful notes. You are ready to call the physician at a moment's notice, if necessary, and to give her emergency assistance as well.

The EEG indicates she is in seizure. High spike waves characteristic of epilepsy appear on the recording. Yet, except for the EEG tracings, your patient appears calm. No lay person would realize that she is having a seizure, or "petit mal," a form of epilepsy which literally means "little sickness."

In just a few brief seconds the seizure is over. Little Lauren, like most people who suffer from petit mal, wasn't even aware that it happened. You ask her how she feels and make more notes. As sometimes happens with a seizure, she says she is sleepy. You let her drift off for just a few minutes while you make more notations for the doctor. You then wake her gently and continue with the exam.

In just a short while the exam is over. As you remove the electrodes and clean her scalp, your young patient demands her reward, and gets it: a small paper finger-puppet made from odds and ends around the EEG lab. She is delighted and wants to know if she can come for another examination. "It was easy," she says.

While Lauren and her mother wait outside, the department chief, Dr. Siraganian, stops in to review her examination. He carefully scans the EEG recordings and asks you to describe Lauren before, during, and immediately after the seizure. Epilepsy, he concludes, is the definite diagnosis. However, Lauren's case is not severe. With simple medication she will lead a completely normal life.

You break for lunch now and join another technologist in the cafeteria. The conversation quickly moves to shop talk. The other technologist can't wait to tell you about his morning in surgery. His patient was undergoing brain surgery in a last attempt to control his violent seizures. All medications had been tried and had failed. Surgery was considered his only hope for a relatively normal life. Before and after surgery your friend monitored the patient's brain waves on the EEG. The change following surgery, he reports, was dramatic.

After lunch you report back to the lab and begin reviewing your next patient's chart, a probable stroke victim. Dr. Siraganian enters the room and your plans for the afternoon abruptly change. We have an "electrocerebral inactivity" case. (The layman's term is brain death.) "I would like you to do it," he says.

You know this will be your last exam for the day, since this test takes several gruelling hours to perform. No technologist likes doing these examinations, particularly when they involve young people. Your case this afternoon will be difficult for just that reason. Your patient, Robert McAndrew, is just thirty years old. A few days earlier he was enjoying the ski slopes. Then a freak accident occurred— not on the slopes but in a car. Like many people today, he has willed his organs to help save another's life in the event of his death. Now the organ transplant team is standing by. All efforts to save the patient have failed. Though his heartbeat is still strong and he is breathing artificially with a respirator, extensive and permanent brain damage has occurred. There is no hope for recovery.

You have performed this examination many times before, efficiently and with no outward emotion, but the experience always leaves a deep impression on you.

You carefully assemble all your equipment and hurry to the patient's floor. The nurse-in-charge briefs you on the patient's condition. There has been no change since the last notation on the patient's records.

Once you are in the room you must decide where to best position your equipment. It is not an easy decision. The EEG will be just one of several pieces of medical equipment in the room. An EKG is recording his heart action; an I.V. (intravenous) bottle is hooked to his arms and legs; tubes run through his nose, while a respirator is keeping his lungs going. Since most of the devices to which he is attached are also electrical, you must be particularly concerned with electrical safety.

The examination itself is the most demanding in your profession. It requires absolute precision and must be done according to very strict procedures. There is no room for errors here. Your hospital and most hospitals today use the Harvard criteria, a special sequence of procedures, to determine brain death. The Harvard criteria require more than just a flat EEG reading to determine brain death. In addition, the patient must be incapable of spontaneous respiration; this means that the patient must not be able to breathe on his own, unassisted by a respirator. Also, no cerebral reflexes of any kind, such as a reaction to sound or light, can be observed.

Precision starts at the very beginning of the exam—when the scalp is cleaned. A much more thorough cleansing than usual is necessary. All possible outside factors which might reduce the machine's ability to pick up electrical brain activity, no matter how slight, must be eliminated.

After his scalp is cleaned, his skull must be measured. While doing this you must be careful not to dislodge any of the tubes in the patient's nose and throat. Extra electrodes are applied to the arms and the legs for this particular examination, similar to the electrode placement on electrocardiograms.

After the last electrode has been attached, you begin checking each to make sure it is properly functioning. When you are absolutely sure everything is working efficiently, the official recording begins.

First you record the brain waves without any outside stimulation. After measuring this recording for about twenty minutes, you are ready for the next part of the examination—the patient's reaction to outside stimulus. You begin by pricking his skin with the needle to observe the EEG reaction to pain. The brain waves remain steady.

You then check for other cerebral reflexes by making noises to test the patient's reaction to sound. You call his name several times. You also lift his eyelids and flash a light in both pupils, again checking for any EEG reactions. The pattern never changes.

Throughout the exam you take notes at each point, recording which stimulus has been used. Nurses come and go, checking the patient's vital signs. Respiratory therapists enter to monitor the respirator. Physicians also drift in and out of the patient's room, constantly checking for changes in his condition. Despite all these interruptions you mustn't be distracted. You must concentrate on the examination at hand.

Finally, after a mentally exhausting three hours, the examination is over. You return to the lab with your results and review the case with the electroencephalographer. Dr. Siraganian confirms that the patient is "dead." Only his body is being kept alive by the machines.

The organ transplant team which has been standing by can now go into action. Soon the patient's body will be prepped and taken to OR for organ removal.

Your day is now officially ended. A life is over, but for those patients who will be receiving Mr. McAndrew's kidneys and eyes, a new life is just beginning.

You joined the technologist for a day. Could you do this job for a lifetime?

PERSONAL QUALIFICATIONS AND WORKING CONDITIONS

There are two important keys to success in this field. The first is the people factor. Since the EEG personnel work with patients on a one-to-one basis all day long, it is extremely important that anyone entering this field not only like patients, but be able to work well with them. This is necessary not only for personal job satisfaction, but in order to perform the work itself. If your feelings aren't positive and genuine you won't have to work long in the field before that is discovered. It will show up on the EEG readings. Patients react to all outside stimulus, particularly that provided by the EEG specialist. As a director of one EEG technology program says, "The technologist's hands are revealing. You can't have cold hands, unfeeling hands whose touch transmits to the patient an 'I'm not concerned about you' attitude." The patient in this kind of atmosphere immediately reacts and the EEG recording produced is less than accurate.

Good observation skills make up the second factor that spells job success in this field. Though as an EEG specialist you are not responsible for EEG interpretation, you must be able to recognize subtle changes in the EEG tracings. With experience, the EEG specialist becomes a master at observation. Some brain seizures, for example, are so subtle that the casual observer and even the patient himself may not realize that one is occurring. The patient may act "strange," but there is no apparent physical problem. The experienced EEG professional must be able to describe in great detail—from start to finish—exactly what has happened. This on-the-scene information is invaluable to the physician for diagnosis.

Generally, working conditions for EEG specialists are good. A forty-hour work week, on a schedule similar to a normal work week, is not uncommon. When one is hospital employed, however, evening and weekend work on a rotating basis may be required. Personnel may also be on call for emergencies.

The job presents no unusual physical demands. Specialists may sit or stand during the examination, depending on the individual circumstances and personal preference. Usually the examination does not require any extensive positioning of the patient, so EEG specialists do not generally have to lift or otherwise physically move patients.

PREPARING FOR TRAINING

Whether you are applying to a technician or a technologist program, a high school education is the first step. Science courses are helpful, particularly biology, since during training you must be able to master basic anatomy and physiology concerning the brain. Courses which will enhance basic math skills are important too. While this career does not involve a great deal of math on the job, you must know how to do simple metric measuring, multiplication, subtraction, division, and percentages. These calculations will be used for determining wave amplitudes, microvolts, millimeters, and other basic EEG control settings.

PROFESSIONAL TRAINING

Courses for the electroencephalographic technician and technologist are given by hospitals, vocational-technical institutes, community colleges, and medical schools. The technician's course lasts for six months; the technologist's, one year. The technician's course is divided into three major elements:

1) *Basic science and clinical pathology,* which are normally encountered in the EEG laboratory. This includes the study of anatomy and physiology of the entire body as it relates to normal brain functioning; physiology and anatomy of the central nervous system, with particular emphasis on the brain; "classic" diseases commonly seen in the laboratory; how to take a patient history for every EEG; and, finally, first aid in the EEG laboratory.

2) *EEG instrumentation.* The basic elements of electricity and electronics that will be needed for EEG operation; concepts such as currents, voltage, and resistance must be understood. Working with plastic models, the student technician also begins to learn the basics of electrical safety.

3) *Basic EEG techniques and clinical experience.* This is the most important part of the student's educational program. Early in the program, usually by the first month, the student is introduced to EEG laboratory procedures. The fundamentals of the normal EEG pattern and the normal variations related to the patient's age and level of consciousness are taught. The student is trained to recognize classic abnormalities in the EEG pattern. Electrode application, the selection

of electrode locations, and different electrode recording sequences—called "montages"—are covered. The student also learns how to make modifications in standard techniques when necessary. Attention is also given to the use of filters and other devices that will improve the accuracy of the reading.

Once basic techniques have been mastered in a simulated setting, the student progresses to actual clinical experience with patients under supervision. In this phase of training, student and teacher work together on a one-to-one basis. Students learn how to work not only within the normal EEG setting, but also under special conditions, such as at the patient's bedside in the intensive care unit and performing basic brain death monitoring.

The clinical work is extensive. Roughly 500 to 600 hours are spent in supervised experience. Throughout this part of the training, the clinical EEGs recorded by the students are reviewed for critical comment by their instructors.

The technologist program covers all the areas just described, but in greater detail. For example, the technician's course in basic techniques may last approximately 20 hours, whereas technologists spend twice the time learning the basics in depth. Principles of laboratory management, including recordkeeping, scheduling, and record storing, are also covered in the technologist's program.

The clinical experience for EEG technologists is more intensive too, and covers a wider range of patient cases. Not only are the more routine EEG cases presented, but students also receive extensive exposure to unusual patient cases. The technologist's education includes a special course which briefly covers clinical medicine, neurology, and neurosurgery. Here the student learns about other diagnostic techniques, such as nuclear medicine, radiography, and electromyography, which are often used in conjunction with the EEG. Student technologists also study briefly the basic principles of psychiatry and behavior, such as basic personality theory and intelligence.

As part of the technologist's course, students are also given a brief introduction to some of the research aspects of the EEG. They attend regular "braincutting" sessions where sections and slices of the human brain are studied microscopically.

Throughout the technologist's course, the emphasis is on educating an EEG specialist who will have both an in-depth and broad knowledge of the field and therefore will be prepared to handle almost any situation.

Programs for both technician and technologist usually award a certificate upon completion. There are a few special two-year college degree programs for the electroencephalographic technologist. The clinical portion of the training is still only one year; however, before entering the year of clinical training, students receive a year of basic sciences and liberal arts courses. Upon completion of the two-year program, students receive the associate degree.

This kind of program offers a strong advantage to students who are interested in teaching, supervisory, and administrative positions. It also gives the student an opportunity to later branch into other allied health fields if he or she so desires. The physician's assistant, registered nursing (at a bachelor's level), physical therapy, and occupational therapy are but a few areas where two years of college or an associate degree are the usual prerequisites. Ultimately, the two-year associate program gives the student the greatest amount of flexibility.

Admissions procedures will vary with each school. In addition to the application form, a personal interview and special admissions test may be required. Students must also show evidence of good health by submitting their own doctor's statement, although in many instances the school provides a physical examination upon acceptance.

Tuition rates are generally low, since many programs are given in community colleges which have low or free tuition. Many hospitals still have a policy of no tuition charge. In addition, stipends and scholarships are often available to help offset the cost of training.

AMA's Committee on Allied Health Education & Accreditation, in cooperation with various professional electroencephalographic associations, accredit programs for the EEG technologist and technician. However, there are many programs which, while not AMA accredited, still provide good education. AMA programs are listed in the school appendix of this book. A list of other recognized schools is available from the American Society of EEG Technologists.

PROFESSIONAL CREDENTIALS

No license is required in this field. Technologists who bear the initials R EEG T after their names have achieved a high degree of competence in their field. These initials mean that they have passed a rigorous written, oral, and practical examination and have become registered electroencephalographic technologists. The examination is given by the American Board of Registration of EEG Technologists. While registration is not a condition for obtaining initial employment, it can be a strong factor in salary increases and job promotions. Technologists who are interested in teaching, administration, or supervisory positions almost always hold the R EEG T.

JOB OPPORTUNITIES

At the present time there is a need for several hundred trained EEG specialists. The field is still considered relatively new and has been growing rapidly with the increased use of the electroencephalograph in surgery, in diagnosing and monitoring patients with brain disease, and in establishing brain death.

According to the U.S. Department of Labor, the employment of the EEG specialists is expected to grow faster than the average for all occupations. The greatest demand, however, will continue to be for the registered EEG technologist.

Hospitals represent the largest employer of EEG personnel, but private EEG laboratories, clinics, and physicians' offices, particularly those specializing in neuro/psychiatric disorders, also offer employment opportunities. While most specialists work with patients in a clinical setting, some also work with physicians and other scientists in research. In this setting much of the work is done with research animals.

Most new graduates of EEG programs find their first jobs through traditional methods—checking local newspapers, contacting hospital personnel officers, or through job listings in the EEG professional journals. Often employers contact schools directly to notify them of available jobs.

Starting salaries vary tremendously depending on the area of the country, the individual employer, and the amount of training the EEG specialist has had. Starting technologists generally earn more than starting technicians. Registered technologists almost always command higher salaries than non-registered technologists. Starting salaries for technologists range approximately in the $8,000 to $11,000 category, with technicians earning slightly less. Experienced technologists can earn upwards of $16,000 to $18,000 or more for advanced teaching, supervising, administration, or research positions.

THE HUMAN SIDE

What attracts people to the EEG field? Each technologist would probably give you a different answer. But Carol Christensen, Education Coordinator of the Presbyterian Hospital School of Electroencephalographic Technology, saw EEG as a unique career opportunity. "I have always been interested in people and medicine. EEG gave me the opportunity to combine both. I didn't have the background to become a doctor and I couldn't spend the number of years necessary in training. But here in the EEG lab I get a chance to work with patients and physicians. I am also involved in the exciting things happening in our brain research department. With just a year of training, I don't think I could have found this kind of combination in another field. I'm here to stay."

For additional information about EEG technology, write:

> American Society of Electroencephalographic Technologists
> 2997 Moon Lake Drive
> West Bloomfield, MI 48033

For additional information on professional credentials, write:

> American Board of Registration of Electroencephalographic
>   Technologists
> EEG-Upham Hall
> University Hospitals
> Columbus, OH 43210

CHAPTER IX

Inside the Surgical Arena

Whether you choose a career in the health field or not, your chances of meeting this health professional at some point in your lifetime are good.

Chances are good, too, that in most cases you won't even remember that the meeting has taken place. Who is this mysterious health professional? The operating room technician.

Today approximately two million operations are performed each year and in almost every case the operating room technician was there, a valued member of the surgical team.

Though surgical history dates back to the Egyptians in 3000 B.C.*, the operating room technician—sometimes called a surgical technician—is a relative newcomer to the surgical scene.

With the expansion of surgical technology in modern medical care, the number of nurses specially trained to assist during surgery could not keep pace with the demand. In 1959, the operating room nurses themselves realized there was a growing need for additional, professionally trained assistants. Through their professional organization, the Association of Operating Room Nurses, the operating room technician was created to fill that gap.

A full ten years passed until, in 1969, the operating room technician gained full professional recognition with the formation of their own professional society, the Association of Operating Room Technicians. On that occasion a message from a founding operating room nurse nicely summed up the technician's new and needed role: "Never before in medical history has there been a greater need for total team work—for all-out team effort. The registered nurse cannot handle the load without the technician; the technician cannot carry more than his or her fair share; and the surgeon is helpless without both."

Surgical technology has advanced rapidly and placed great demands on the surgical team. Operations such as heart transplants, which were only dreamed about years ago, are now commonplace realities. But whether routine or not, the success of any operation depends on the teamwork of all the surgical staff—physicians, nurses, and operating room technicians. Each team member works with different responsibilities to insure that each patient receives the best surgical care possible.

---

* Egyptians bored holes in the skull to release "evil spirits."

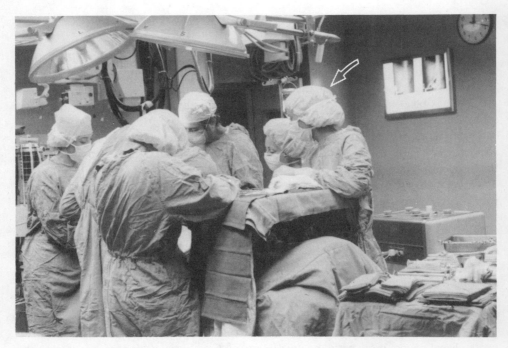

During surgery the surgeon, anesthesiologist, circulators, and scrubs must all work together as one. Arrow shows the scrub technician. Courtesy of Debbra Dunning, Welborn Baptist Hospital.

MEET THE SURGICAL TEAM

Inside the surgical arena you will encounter others beside the patient and surgeon. Working with the surgeon is the anesthesiologist, another physician who has received special, additional training in the use of anesthesia. The anesthesiologist's role is equally important to that of the surgeon. Despite the surgeon's skill, an operation cannot be successfully performed if the patient is not made completely insensible to pain. Administering anesthesia itself is more complicated than just administering a gas or simple injection. It is a highly complex physiological process which requires constant monitoring on the part of the anesthesiologist to insure that the patient suffers no harmful reaction as a result of these powerful medications.

In some instances the person administering the anesthesia may be a nurse—the nurse anesthetist. This is a registered nurse who has received two years of intensive special training in anesthesia and works with patient cases which are generally less complicated.

In addition to the anesthesiologist or nurse anesthetist, first and second surgical assistants are usually also present. Second assistants are usually medical students who are learning the basics of surgical medicine through direct observation within the operating room. First assistants are more than passive observers. To some extent, they participate in the simpler aspects of surgery. First assistants are usually residents, doctors who have graduated from medical school but are still in training. Sometimes first assistants are physician's assistants, a new allied health profession closely related to medicine. Finally there are the nurses and operating room technicians, who work closely together to assist the surgeon during the operation.

GENERAL RESPONSIBILITIES

The operating room technician plays an active role before, during, and after surgery. Though specific job responsibilities may vary with the employer, the technician has been specially trained to assist in a wide variety of surgical tasks.

Before surgery can be performed, a great deal of preparation is required. The patient, operating room, and surgical staff must all be ready.

Patient preparation involves several steps and begins long before the patient reaches the operating room.

One important part of the "prep" (hospital jargon for presurgical patient preparation) requires that the operative site be made as germfree as possible. This is a two-step process. First the operative area must be washed, shaved, and disinfected, either the night before or several hours before the actual operation begins. A second, simpler disinfecting of the area takes place immediately before surgery.

Depending on the policy of the individual hospital where the technician works, the technician may be responsible for both processes. In some hospitals the nursing staff may do the first, more extensive cleansing. In the operating room area itself, the technician positions the patient, carries out the second prepping, and drapes the surgical area with sterile sheets.

The patient preparation is only one phase of preoperative procedures and of the technician's responsibility. The operating room must be fully equipped for the surgery that will take place. This again is the technician's job. Every instrument that the surgeon might need during the operation must be properly assembled. Every suture, sponge, or other surgical supportive device must be on hand. Any special fluids that the patient might require, such as blood, plasma, or saline (a simple salt solution), must be ready and immediately available. Lights must be adjusted, equipment positioned; no detail of the operation can escape the technician's eyes or be left to chance.

Like the patient, the surgical team must also be fully prepared for the surgery. Wherever possible, the threat of infection must be eliminated. Anyone entering the operating room must first undergo germ "decontamination" procedures. Street clothes must be exchanged for sterile hospital gowns or suits; hair must be covered with a special cap; hands must be thoroughly washed and gloved.

Just how extensive the required procedures are depends on the responsibility each person assumes during surgery. Anyone in the area immediately surrounding the patient and the operating room table, called the operating field, must adhere to the strictest measures—they must be "sterile." Those working outside this area but still within the operating room must follow careful but less stringent procedures.

During the operation itself the technician acts in one of two principal assisting roles: as a scrub or a circulator. As the "scrub," the technician is teamed directly with the surgeon and acts as an extension of the surgeon's hands. A scrub is responsible for handing the surgeon any and all instruments, sponges, sutures, or any other materials that he or she needs to perform the operation. The scrub also removes used sponges and other items from the operating field, passing them to the circulator.

The circulator's role is different. Circulators act as the legs of the operating room staff, constantly "circulating" through the surgical arena, adjusting lights, restocking surgical supplies and insuring that any additional items which the surgeons may need, such as medication, will be immediately at hand. In addition, circulators receive the used sponges or any other materials passed by the scrub. Before the operation can be considered officially over, each sponge and instrument must be counted as a control check to guard against any objects becoming accidentally left in the patient. Blood-soaked sheets, towels, and sponges must also be weighed and the remaining blood and transfusion bottles measured to determine the patient's blood loss during the operation.

But even when work as a scrub or circulator is done, and the operation is officially over, the operating room technician's job is not ended.

Technicians may assist in transferring the patient to a stretcher en route to the recovery room. Then the operating room must be cleaned up, used articles must be collected and discarded or, if reusable, sterilized and repacked into new surgical sets and stored away. Then the operating room must be carefully set up for the next case. There may be other work too, such as ordering out-of-stock supplies and simple department recordkeeping.

WORKING ON THE TEAM

Though the amount of patient contact operating room technicians have varies from hospital to hospital, they generally do work with some patients person-to-person. They also have a great deal of contact with the rest of the surgical team. Good operating room procedures require operating room technicians to work closely together with all other team members for the good of the patient. Each person must be depended upon to meet his or her own responsibilities.

Contact is generally divided between doctors and nurses. When scrubbing, the technician works on a one-to-one basis with the surgeon; when circulating, close physician contact is with the anesthesiologist.

The OR technician works with registered nurses who often act as supervisors or circulators. Though not all OR supervisors are registered nurses (some are operating room technicians), the majority are. Many circulators are also RNs.

Whether the technician is assigned as a circulator or as a scrub depends on the individual hospital's policy. It may seem surprising, but the circulator's role is considered the more demanding one in the operating room, despite the fact that he or she does not work directly with the surgeon. The reason for this is that the circulator has the responsibility of insuring that everything the surgeon may need for the operation, whether it be medication, blood, electrical equipment, or anything else, is immediately on hand. Circulators, as the surgeon's supply line, must constantly assess what is happening in the operating room so that they can anticipate what will be needed. Often an RN and an operating room technician (ORT) are teamed and work as a circulating pair, although two technicians may work together as well in the same capacity if hospital policy permits.

INSIDE THE SURGICAL ARENA

The best way to understand what happens inside the surgical arena is to work there. So put yourself inside this operating room suite and behind the surgical mask.

It's your first scrub of the day and it is not quite 8 A.M. You have already exchanged your civilian clothes for your operating room scrub attire, which is provided by the hospital. Your outfit, while not fashionable, is essential to asepsis (meaning free from bacteria and other micro-organisms) within the OR. This clothing must be kept as germfree as possible and is worn only while inside the surgical area. From head to toe you are specially dressed—from the scrub cap that completely covers your hair to your special Scandinavian clogs which are grounded for electrical safety and encased in shoe covers to reduce germ contamination. Before you start your scrub, you don your surgical mask, carefully making sure it covers your nose and mouth without gapping at the sides.

Before you begin the last step in your ritual, the scrub, you check with Ms. Jones, another certified operating room technician (CORT). She is a circulator for this morning's operation. "All set up?" you ask. "We're fine," she replies. There are two circulators assigned this morning, so no additional help is needed to set up. You can now begin your scrub. As a scrub technician, you, like the surgeon and any other team members in the immediate operating field, must be as clean as the surgical clothes you are wearing.

You begin the process. Your hospital follows a timed ten-minute scrub procedure. The scrubbing, while not a complicated procedure, requires care. Despite the fact that you have done this hundreds of times before, you must do it methodically, overlooking no detail. You must scrub all surfaces of the hands and arms to three inches above the elbow. There can be no shortcuts in this process. Infection is one of the biggest threats of any operation. Strict rules in the OR focus on preventing and minimizing this patient hazard.

You start by simply washing your hands and then meticulously scraping under each fingernail with a pointed nail file. Then, using a small brush, you begin scrubbing your left hand, using a firm motion and an ample supply of antiseptic solution, and rinsing frequently. The wall clock tells you a full minute has passed. You can now move to the next area. One minute more and you can proceed from the arm to the elbow. One half minute. Rinse. Brush. Then the ritual begins again, this time with the right hand. Once your hands are initially scrubbed, you hold them higher than your elbows to prevent any water from running back. This water would contribute to germ growth. Then the process starts again. This time you can eliminate the elbow scrub. Four more minutes of scrubbing, and you wind up with a half-minute scrub on each hand. You turn the faucet using your elbow, careful to avoid any hand contact with the knob, which would spoil your efforts. Sterile towels are nearby for drying. Your hands, now surgically clean, are still not sterile. Despite this extensive scrubbing, only half the bacteria population has been eliminated. Ms. Jones enters to assist you with gowning and gloving.

You enter the operating room and begin preparing the back table "setup" for today's operation: exploratory abdominal surgery. You remove the necessary items from the sterile supply case and begin assembling the table: surgeon's gowns, patient's drapes, dissecting scissors, thumb forceps, retractors, sponges, Kelley clamps, towel clips, extra scalpels, sterile paper bags for suture wrappers, needle holders, and suction tips. After this back table has been set up, you prepare the

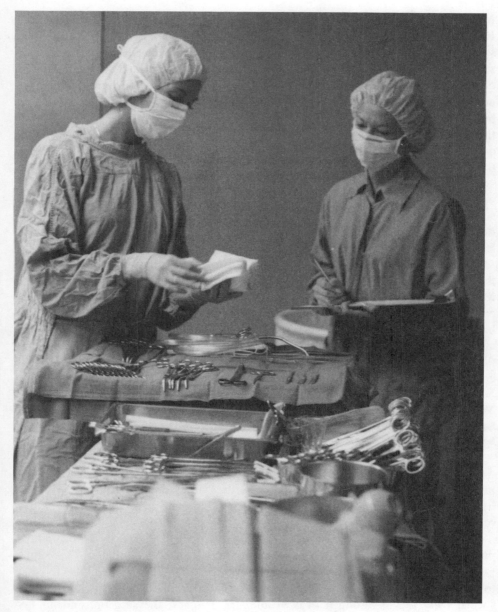

In the OR, needles and sponges are counted and recounted by a CORT with the supervision of a circulator. Courtesy of Debbra Dunning, Welborn Baptist Hospital.

Mayo tray, which will contain the items that the surgeon will immediately need. Reels of suture, retractors, sponges, suture scissors, clamps, thumb forceps, and scalpels are among the items you place on the tray. Because this is exploratory surgery, there is no way of predicting what the surgeon will find, so you must have on hand special instruments in addition to the basic abdominal setup. When you are finished you have assembled almost 150 separate items—not just in any fashion, but in a neat, highly organized manner. Each item must be in the proper place so that you can pass it to the surgeon without a moment's hesitation. You carefully double-check your instruments and supplies against the surgeon's check list. Everything is there and in order.

You are now ready to begin the count of sponges, needles, and instruments. This is always done with two persons, a scrub and a circulator. Each checks the other so there will be no chance of error. This will be done three times before the operation is officially over. Every item must be accounted for. A sponge or other object left in the patient accidentally could prove fatal.

While you and the other circulator—Ms. Shogan, a registered nurse—conduct the count, Ms. Jones wheels the patient into the OR. Following proper procedure, Ms. Jones reviews his chart. She checks to see if the operative permit has been correctly signed; if the laboratory reports are complete; if pre-operative medications have been given as ordered; and if the patient has been properly prepared. She also carefully checks the patient's identification, by checking his hospital identification band and then asking the patient his name. Though he is groggy, he is still conscious. "Moscone," he responds to her question.

Now, with Ms. Jones assisting, the anesthesiologist administers the anesthesia. Mr. Moscone squeezes her hand tightly. Like many patients, he is anxious and a bit frightened. She holds his hand and speaks to him reassuringly. In just a few seconds he has lost consciousness.

He is then positioned for surgery. Even this seemingly small detail requires precision on the ORT's part. The patient will be in the operating position for several hours and if he is improperly positioned, serious nerve damage could result. Once he is positioned, Ms. Jones completes a second surgical prep. The patient is now ready for draping.

This aspect, and many others that will follow, will give you an opportunity to put into action your knowledge of anatomy and surgical techniques. This simple procedure requires you to know what kind of incision the surgeon will use in order to properly drape the patient. Once finished, Mr. Moscone is entirely covered with sheets. Only the operating field is visible. Dr. Hughes, the surgeon, and his first assistant, Dr. Pine, a new resident, enter. You help them gown and glove. Everything is ready to begin. Everyone moves to the operating field. "Scalpel," Dr. Hughes says. You hand him the instrument; the operation is officially underway.

Dr. Hughes is particularly quick. Working with each surgeon is different. Each has a particular surgical rhythm. The patient, too, makes a difference in the operation. Each person's physical characteristics and clinical condition are unique.

Throughout the operation you not only continue to supply Dr. Hughes with the instruments he requests, but you anticipate his needs by applying your knowledge of surgery where possible. When he calls for a scalpel or scissors, you know that clamps will most likely be needed next. When clamps are used, sutures may be necessary. Each item is handed to the surgeon deftly, in such a way that it can be immediately used. While the operation is in progress, your concentration is unbroken. You keep your eyes and ears open, listening attentively to everything Dr. Hughes says and watching the operation closely so you can stay one jump ahead of him. Periodically he asks you to cut a suture or calls for suction. You remove blood-soaked sponges and pass them to Ms. Jones.

Meanwhile, she and the circulator nurse are busy keeping the operating room neat, making sure equipment and supplies are on hand and that aseptic technique is being maintained at all times. The anesthesiologist requests a drug. Ms. Jones leaves the area to retrieve it.

Dr. Hughes is finally inside the abdominal cavity. He removes a small piece of tissue from what appears to be a small tumor. Using forceps you pass the specimen to Ms. Shogan who, in turn, places it in a small container, labels it carefully, and sends it to the pathologist. In the pathologist's laboratory it will be analyzed immediately while Dr. Hughes waits. The pathologist's report will supply Dr. Hughes with critical information on how extensive the rest of the surgery must be. Within minutes the report is back. "Benign," Ms. Jones reports. Mr. Moscone is lucky; the tumor is not cancerous.

You feel beads of perspiration gathering on your forehead. Ms. Jones has already noticed too and blots them away. You cannot perform this simple task yourself. It would be a break in aseptic technique.

Before Dr. Hughes closes the abdominal cavity, you and the circulator again do a count of all the items used in the operation. This is repeated again just before the skin is closed. Everything is accounted for. Dr. Hughes asks Dr. Pine to close. Even though the incision is closed, you leave your surgical table set up. An emergency can still arise even at this point of the operation, and these items could still be needed. The anesthesiologist gives the go-ahead. The patient can now be removed to the recovery room.

Now that the patient is gone, the operation officially is over. You and Ms. Jones begin cleaning up the operating room. The linen on the operating room table is removed and the table is washed with disinfectant solution. Refuse from the wastebasket and kickbuckets is removed; nondisposable sponges are put in the laundry. Suction equipment is cleaned and readied for the next procedure. Finally, the floor is damp-mopped with disinfectant. You change gowns and get ready for the next procedure.

The rest of the day goes quickly. Your next scrub is for a minor surgical procedure, and after lunch you spend the afternoon working as a circulator. Finally, at 3:30, the day is over—at least you hope so. You are "on call" tonight, so you never know what the evening will hold.

Now that you have gotten a brief glimpse of life within the operating room, could your future hold a spot on a surgical team?

PERSONAL QUALIFICATIONS AND WORKING CONDITIONS

The work environment of the operating room is unique and makes special demands on those choosing this career. There are no coffee breaks or rest periods, no time off between periods of peak work activities. The operating room demands complete concentration. No operation can ever be considered routine and you must constantly be prepared for the unexpected.

To work successfully within this kind of environment, the technician needs important basic qualifications:

* An ability to function well under stress, which is a part of the everyday work environment;

* An ability to think quickly and respond to the surgeon's demands;

* Good manual dexterity;

* Finally, good organization and an eye for detail, in order to properly set up the operating room equipment and surgical supplies.

The profession is physically demanding, not in terms of sheer physical strength, but in stamina. To put it plainly, it requires leg work, whether the technician works as a scrub, standing in one spot for several hours assisting the surgeon, or as a circulator, standing and moving about the operating room as required.

Work hours may be irregular too. Most hospital schedules require technicians to work a rotating shift, and there may be night time or on-call emergency duty as well. Usually a hospital operates between two and four shifts during an operating room day, although a few hospitals may operate around the clock. In a large medical center, a four-shift day might run: 7:30 A.M.–4:00 P.M., 10:00 A.M.–7:00 P.M., 4:00 P.M.–12:00 midnight or 12:00 noon–8:00 P.M., followed by the on-call period. Technicians working in this institution might have a work schedule of three days per week on the 7:30 A.M.–4:00 P.M. shift and two days a week on the 10:00 A.M.–7:00 P.M. shift, with "on-call" scheduled as well. In a small hospital, the operating room staff might work fairly regular 7:30 A.M.–4:00 P.M. workdays with on-call work for emergencies only.

PREPARING FOR THE PROFESSION

Before you can apply to a school of operating room technology, you must hold a high school diploma or its equivalent. Each program sets its own specific entrance requirements. A student who has followed a general high school curriculum which has included some laboratory science, particularly biology, would fulfill the entrance requirements of most operating room technician programs.

Though the profession itself is demanding, this is one technological profession where extensive science and math preparation are not required. Little math is used on the job itself except for simple measurements, sponge and instrument counts, and calculating blood loss. Biology is the fundamental prerequisite science needed for operating room technology. This will help you to master basic microbiology, anatomy, physiology, and pathology during operating room training. Many students find that additional science and math courses, though not required, serve them well later, should they decide to branch into other technological careers.

PROFESSIONAL TRAINING

The training is fast-paced, ranging from as little as a nine-month certificate program to a two-year community college associate degree program. Certificate programs are offered by hospitals, vocational-technical institutes, and community colleges. However, only a community college can award a two-year associate degree in operating room technology.

The training itself covers both classroom and clinical work. To work well as an operating room technologist, one must have a basic knowledge of anatomy, physiology, and pathology. The OR technician must understand what is happening on the operating room table. Microbiology is another basic science which is extremely important, since micro-organisms pose a constant threat of infection to the patient.

In addition to these basic sciences the student receives an orientation to the operating room covering medical terminology, medical legal aspects of surgery, the ethics of the hospital, and basic weights and measurements, and is introduced to the operating room environment.

The student OR technician also learns the fundamentals of safe patient care, how to transport patients, the basics of anesthesia, and patient positioning. Related nursing procedures, such as skin preparation and environmental control during the operation, are also taught.

Finally, operating room techniques and surgical procedures must be thoroughly covered. In this phase of training, the student learns about sterilization and disinfection, preparation and care of surgical supply and equipment, proper aseptic technique and the responsibilities of the technician as circulating or scrub assistant.

In addition to general surgery, the student studies specialized surgical procedures used in obstetrics and gynecology, ophthalmology, plastic surgery, oral surgery, orthopedic surgery, and neurosurgery, to name just a few areas. Each of these surgical areas may use a variation of instruments, needles, sutures, and sponges. The student must learn the basic surgical setup for each.

But the only way a student can learn all this is through supervised clinical experience. Student OR technicians get plenty. For example, in the nine-month program at Columbia Presbyterian Medical Center in New York City, more than half the student's time is spent in clinical experience.

The introduction to clinical work comes early. It has to in a nine- to twelve-month program. Students begin their clinical experience by observing in the operating room. But soon, within as little as two months after training begins, they begin scrubbing and assisting the surgeon with minor surgery. As clinical training advances, students become more experienced and will rotate through several surgical areas. Generally two to three weeks is spent on a specialized surgical area, such as orthopedics. However, true competence in a specialized surgical area requires at least four to five months of intensive work experience. So an essential part of the ORT's education really comes after training is completed. School simply gives the student a basic foundation upon which later work experience builds.

An associate degree program operates a little differently, since this is a two-year program. Students study basic sciences and liberal arts courses in addition to the clinical and surgical courses already described. However, they also go through the rigorous clinical work experience, usually starting in the first semester with observing in the operating room. Prior to getting actual work experience in an operating room at an affiliated hospital, students learn in a simulated campus setting. For example, at Nassau County (N.Y.) Community College there is a completely equipped OR right on the campus. Here students in a nonstressful environment learn the techniques which will later be required in the operating room.

An associate degree program offers many advantages. The first is college credits, which can later be applied to other allied health areas, should a student decide he or she wishes to go on for further education. Many of the graduates of the Nassau County Community program have done just that—going on to get bachelor's degrees in nursing or physicians assisting. They were able to do this because they already had to their credit the two years of college which is generally required for admission to these programs.

Class sizes in both certificate and associate degree programs vary; generally, they range from 8 to 30 students. Competition for admission to training varies also. A college program, in general, is more competitive. In addition to a transcript of your high school record, personal recommendations, a physical examination, and, in some cases, an entrance examination are required before you may be accepted to hospital or college programs. Many programs also require a personal interview, which helps determine if the student is really interested and motivated enough to enter this field.

If cost is a factor in determining whether you can train for this profession, you should be reassured by the fact that most programs charge little or no tuition. College programs, however, are the exception to this rule. They charge tuition that is comparable to other school programs. Another totally free educational route exists within operating room technology—training within the military. The Army, Air Force, and Navy conduct training programs in operating room technology, with the Navy course generally rated number one.

PROFESSIONAL CREDENTIALS

The initials CORT after a technician's name indicate superiority in this field. Those who become certified operating room technicians have proven their expertise by successfully completing a 250-question examination. The exam, which is sponsored by the Association of Operating Room Technicians (AORT), covers all aspects of operating room technology: basic sciences, safe patient care, aseptic technique and environmental control, supplies and equipment, and surgical procedures. The examination is developed with the assistance of OR educators—surgeons, nurses, and technicians throughout the country. To be eligible to sit for the examination, in general, a technician must have graduated from a military, accredited, or otherwise AORT-approved program. Students who will graduate prior to the examination date are also eligible. In some instances, experience or current employment is required.

Though certification is not an absolute requirement for employment, it is always preferred. This is understandable, because the initials CORT tell a perspective employer that a technician has a broad general knowledge of operating room technology and the ability to apply it properly. At present there is no licensure in this field, so certification is strongly relied on by employers to insure competency.

JOB OPPORTUNITIES

What is the employment outlook for ORTs? Good. And likely to remain so through the mid-1980's, particularly for the certified ORT. In fact, the need for these workers should double within the next ten years. Among the factors which contribute to this favorable employment outlook are the growth in population, the greater ability of people to pay for surgery through prepaid medical plans, and ever-improving procedures and surgical techniques which contribute to greater surgical success. These factors have created an increased demand for surgical services. Currently, about 60% of all patients entering hospitals enter as surgical patients.

Other trends within surgical technology are affecting the role of the operating room technician as well. The number of OR registered nurses is decreasing and many ORTs are now taking over, more routinely, the circulating role. In some special instances, where hospital policies and the individual surgeon permit the role of the ORT has been expanded to that of acting as a first assistant.

Hospitals remain the largest single employer, but even within hospitals, employment opportunities are varied. ORTs are employed in emergency room and delivery room, as well as in traditional OR settings. In addition, some technicians work as private assistants, working for a single surgeon or for a practicing group of six to twelve surgeons.

Considering the length of training, usually one year or less, starting salaries are good, too. A starting technician can expect to earn about $9,000 to $11,000, depending upon where the job is located and whether he or she is certified. With advancement and greater experience within the field, salaries increase, along with job responsibilities. With additional training and experience, operating room technicians may advance to supervisory or teaching positions. Some technicians also advance by working in highly specialized areas, such as ophthalmic or open heart surgery.

DO YOU CLICK?

What draws a person to this field? How do you know that it is for you? One experienced CORT gave this as her reason for joining the profession: "What attracted me to the field was that the work is fast-paced and continuous. Though there is a definite routine that must be strictly followed, to me the work itself is never routine. It is always interesting because I am involved with my cases. I also like the science side. I get to see living anatomy. The human body, indeed, is a fascinating machine. But the operating room is not a place for everyone. You must 'click' with it immediately. Some people say it's too impersonal, but that's not the way I see it. Though I am not always involved with the patient on a one-to-one basis, I still care."

For additional information on operating room technology and professional credentials, write:

> The Association of Operating Room Technicians
> 1100 West Littleton Boulevard, Suite 201
> Littleton, CO 80120

CHAPTER X

The Life Machine

Working inside you right now is one of the most efficient filtering systems known—your kidneys. Each day these remarkable organs filter about 200 quarts of blood through your body, ridding it of excess fluid and waste products, retaining necessary body fluids and chemicals and releasing into your bloodstream vital hormones that help control your blood pressure and production.

Yet, for all their important work, nature's built-in filters are amazingly compact. Together your kidneys weigh less than a pound and each is no larger than your fist.

Lose one kidney and little is changed. Your remaining kidney enlarges slightly, increases its efficiency by 50%, and normal healthy life continues. But lose both kidneys and your life hangs in the balance. Fluids build up in body tissues; dangerous waste products collect in the bloodstream, and without their removal life slips away in about a week's time.

Until the early 1960's, this was the fate of some 100,000 Americans each year. Without organ transplantation, kidney failure was always fatal.

Biomedical technology changed that desperate situation with the development of the dialysis machine, which artificially removes waste products from the blood. Todays, thanks to dialysis, over 36,000 patients are being kept alive even though their kidneys no longer function. Truly, the dialysis machine is a life machine.

A NEW HEALTH PROFESSION EMERGES

With the advent of dialysis came new life for patients and new jobs for those who cared for them. Initially physicians and nurses were the major health professionals involved in dialysis care. Patients were plentiful but the machines available were few—only 750 people were on dialysis in 1967. By 1969, however, this number had more than tripled. Additional qualified personnel were needed to assist with the complicated dialysis procedure. Thus the dialysis technician was born.

Slowly the dialysis field began to grow. But before the field could really blossom, one major obstacle remained—money. Though technology and personnel were now available to accommodate patients needing dialysis care, few patients, even those with medical insurance, could afford it. Generally only the wealthy, with limitless pocketbooks, or the poor, whose medical bill could be paid through the

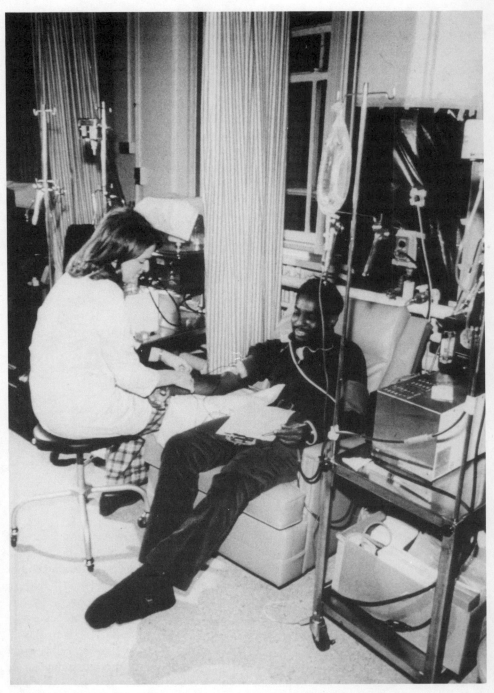

Dialysis technician prepares patient for treatment in an outpatient dialysis clinic. Courtesy of National Kidney Foundation.

federal government's Medicaid program, could meet the $10,000 to $50,000-a-year price that dialysis care demanded.

In November 1972, this situation changed dramatically when a special law amending the Social Security Act was passed. The new law provided Medicare coverage for most persons requiring dialysis treatment, irrespective of age. Under this Medicare program, 80% of all dialysis costs would be borne by the federal government.

Since this legislation was passed, the number of persons receiving dialysis care, the facilities where it is available, and the number of personnel who provide care have grown rapidly. In addition to physicians and administrative manpower, an estimated 10,000 to 12,000 persons are employed in dialysis care. Of these, approximately 25% are dialysis technicians; the rest are registered nurses.

A MEMBER OF THE TEAM

Good dialysis care depends on teamwork among physicians, nurses, and technicians. Each member of the team plays a different but interrelated role.

Heading the team is the nephrologist or renal physician, a doctor specializing in kidney disorders. He or she is responsible for the patient's overall health care and for prescribing a treatment plan. While a person is on dialysis, myriad health problems can and often do occur. Consequently, constant medical supervision is extremely important.

The nephrology nurse, a registered nurse, has many different responsibilities. They can be summed up as developing and supervising the treatment which is prescribed by the physician. This includes more than just the actual dialysis treatment itself. The treatment plan focuses on all aspects of the patient's care, including the prescribed diet, medication, exercise and physical activity, and the patient's psychological and social adjustments to his or her illness. In some dialysis treatment units nurses perform dialysis procedures. In other units RNs only act as supervisors.

Finally, working under the supervision of the nephrology nurse, the dialysis technician provides the extra hands for the technical support of dialysis work within the unit.

Because this profession is still in its infancy, job duties for dialysis technicians are not standardized across the country, but vary from employer to employer. In some dialysis units technicians may work more as biomedical equipment technicians, maintaining and repairing equipment and performing general support duties. In other units technicians with advanced education and experience may be responsible for nearly all aspects of the dialysis program. In general, though, most technicians work between these two extremes, performing basic dialysis patient care duties and machine maintenance.

Their job involves a great deal of responsibility. During dialysis, the patient's life depends on the treatment going properly. The technician is there to make sure that this is exactly what happens.

You can better understand the technician's job if you know something about dialysis itself.

HOW DIALYSIS WORKS

Dialysis itself is the process of maintaining the chemical balance of the blood when the kidneys have failed. In hemodialysis, "hemo" meaning blood, the patient's blood must circulate outside the body. (Thus it is a form of extracorporeal technology, meaning outside the body.) The blood is taken from a blood vessel in the arm or the leg by a needle inserted into the blood vessel. The needle is attached to a tube which carries the patient's blood to the artificial kidney machine. The patient's heart pumps blood through the tube to the machine. Here impurities from the blood pass through a dialysis membrane, which is made of cellophane and shaped like a tube.

The patient's blood is inside the tube; on the outside is a chemical bath called the "dialysate." As the blood comes into contact with the inside of the dialysis membrane, certain waste products, which are dissolved in high concentration in the blood, pass through or "diffuse" through the membrane into the dialysate. Then the dialysate, which now contains these waste products, is washed away by fresh dialysate solution. This process is continuous and eliminates the waste products from the body.

But this is only one part of the dialysis process. While waste products are being removed from the blood, substances which the body needs and which the dialysate contains, such as calcium or dextrose, also pass from the dialysate through the membrane into the blood. Once this two-way exchange has occurred, the blood is returned to the patient's body through another tube that is connected to a different vein by a needle.

During the dialysis process, osmosis* also occurs. Excess fluids flow into the dialysis bath. With the addition of a pump to the hemodialysis machine, additional fluids are removed through ultrafiltration. These three processes—diffusion, osmosis, and ultrafiltration—all occur simultaneously.

Though most people don't realize it, another form of dialysis exists—peritoneal dialysis. This dialysis is used much less frequently than hemodialysis. Peritoneal dialysis also requires a special machine; but in this dialysis the peritoneum, the membrane which surrounds the patient's intestines and other abdominal organs, is used instead of artificial cellophane tubing.

---

* Osmosis: The passage of fluid through a membrane separating solutions of varying concentrations. The fluid passes through the membrane from the region of lower concentration of dissolved substance to the region of higher concentration of a dissolved substance. The two solutions tend to reach equal concentrations.

The dialysate is introduced directly into the abdominal cavity through a tube and floods the entire peritoneal membrane. Diffusion and osmosis then take place, removing the waste products and excess fluids. After the two-way exchange occurs, the dialysate is drained from the abdomen. This cycle of flooding and draining is repeated many times until the patient's entire blood supply has been dialyzed.

Though both systems may appear simple in theory, they are highly technical processes. Performing and monitoring this technical process is the primary role of the dialysis technician.

THE DIALYSIS TECHNICIAN AND PATIENT

The patients may be any age, any background, but they all have one thing in common—kidney failure. Most are the victims of chronic kidney failure, in which the kidneys falter and slowly lose their ability to function over a period of several years. Finally, when a carefully controlled diet and drugs can no longer compensate for the loss of kidney function and only 5 to 10% of their kidney function remains, they enter "end stage renal disease." At this point only a transplant or dialysis can save their lives. A few lucky ones suffer acute kidney failure. This is kidney failure which occurs suddenly, often as a result of poisoning, drug overdoses, multiple body injuries from car accidents, a kidney blockage, or other kidney problems. These patients are lucky because, in most cases, the kidney failure is only temporary. Dialysis is just an interim measure which keeps them alive until their kidney function is restored naturally within a few weeks.

Technicians work with patients suffering from both types of kidney failure. Generally those with chronic failure are treated in out-patient E.S.R.S. facilities (end stage renal disease) which may operate as a hospital clinic or an independent dialysis care facility. Those chronically ill patients who are too sick at the outset of treatment, have serious medical complications, or will be undergoing surgery, are hospitalized, as are those who are suffering from acute kidney failure. Since these in-hospital cases are generally more complex, a technician working with these patients must have topnotch skills.

But whether working with in-patients or out-patients, the technician's job is basically the same: to perform the dialysis treatment with the highest level of patient care and safety.

Because the machine and patient are "one" in dialysis, united by a common blood supply, the technician's responsibility cannot be divorced from either.

The preparation of the machine, both before and after, is critical. The dialysate must be properly mixed, the machine properly primed and set up. Whatever enters the machines ultimately enters the patient's body, so there is no margin for error. After the treatment, the machine must be thoroughly cleaned and sterilized. This minimizes the risk of bacterial infection and hepatitis (a serious disease of the liver) which are ever-present threats in the dialysis unit.

During treatment, the machine and the patient must be carefully monitored. If the machine malfunctions during treatment, the patient will immediately be affected. The patient must also be constantly observed. Some malfunctions are apparent only through changes in the patient.

The dialysis technician, perhaps more than most other health professionals, develops close ties with the patients. Understandably, they are linked by time. No other health professional, whether doctor or social worker or supervising nurse, usually spends as much time with the patient as the dialysis technician. Each hemodialysis treatment takes four to five hours to complete, and most patients require two to four dialysis sessions per week. This pattern continues not just for several weeks but throughout the patient's lifetime. This brings the technician in close contact with much more than just the medical aspects of the patient's life. The patient's family, friends, and work become a part of the technician's life too.

There are other psychological ties as well. During treatment the patient is fully dependent on the technician's skills. The technician, as well as the machine, is the patient's lifeline. Like the machine, the patient requires care before, during, and after dialysis treatment, which the technician provides.

The dialysis technician is intimately involved with the patient. You need only spend a few hours in a dialysis unit to see why.

INSIDE A DIALYSIS UNIT

It is dinnertime. Traffic is starting to pick up; you are one of the travelers, too. Only you are not going home, like most motorists—you are heading for work in a dialysis unit.

You are working the late shift this week. Many of your patients will be coming to the Center after they have completed their day's work.

When you arrive at the Center, you change into your white lab coat and then check the schedule of patients whom you will be seeing this evening. Tonight you will be working with three patients. You carefully check all the supplies that you will need and then head to the supply room for a few missing odds and ends.

As soon as you return to the dialysis unit, you begin carefully checking the dialysis machine that you will be using for your first patient, Mr. Klopp. You assemble all the necessary supplies and tubing for the dialysis procedure, and then mix the dialysis solution which will be used. This step requires great care. A solution which contains the wrong amount of potassium or other substances could cause a severe reaction in the patient. For this reason your machine has many different monitoring devices and safety alarms which will immediately signal a chemical imbalance in the dialysis bath, should this occur. You carefully mix the concentrated chemicals with purified water, hook up the machine, and then carefully test for machine leaks. All systems seem "go," so you begin to prime the dialyzer with your fluid. This also is extremely important. All air must be removed from the machine and the tubing, since any air present will be pumped into the patient, causing death. As soon as you are satisfied that the machine is set up properly, you are ready for your patient.

Mr. Klopp has just arrived. By now you two are old friends. He has been coming to the Center four times a week over the past two years. The change in him during this period has been dramatic. When he initially came to the unit he was extremely depressed about his condition. He worried constantly about whether or not he could continue working and supporting his family. During those first few weeks of treatment he needed special care, attention, and encouragement. It has paid off. He has been able to continue working days by participating in this evening dialysis program.

Before you begin the actual dialysis treatment you take his vital signs— temperature, pulse, respiration—and note them carefully in his patient chart. You also weigh the patient, another standard procedure. He has gained a little over four pounds since his last visit. You begin questioning him closely about his diet. A four-pound gain is not much in a normal person whose kidneys are functioning, but they can be critical to a dialysis patient. This signals that a fluid overload is building up. Unlike a normal person, a dialysis patient produces little or no urine, the body's way of ridding itself of excess water and salt. Salt and water enter the body chiefly through diet. Therefore, a dialysis patient's diet must be controlled to the smallest detail. An extra Coke or a glass of water is a forbidden luxury to the dialysis patient. Dialysis can remove only three pounds of fluid, so it will leave Mr. Klopp with an additional pound. If this continues to build over a period of time, his heart will become overtaxed. Symptoms such as shortness of breath and swelling of the ankles will occur. If the overload is not corrected, your patient will be in serious trouble. You remind him about fluid overload and explain that the easiest way to deal with this problem is to avoid it. He promises to be more careful about his diet and you make a special note on his chart.

You carefully inspect the place on his arm where the dialysis needle will be inserted. It looks good. No sign of soreness. You carefully clean the skin and apply an antiseptic. Your patient will be connected to the machine by an "internal fistula," which is an artificial connection made between an artery and a vein underneath the skin. The fistula is created through minor surgery. Before this method was perfected, patients were connected to the machine by means of external tubes. These external "shunts," still used in some cases, require great care. Infections are a constant problem and there is always the danger that their tubes may pull out. The internal fistula is always preferred. It requires no special care between dialysis treatments and there is no danger of its coming loose. You carefully apply novocaine to the skin and then insert the sterile needle painlessly. Mr. Klopp's blood is soon filtering through the tubes connected to the machine.

To prevent the blood from clotting during dialysis, you have added an anti-coagulant (meaning "against clotting") called heparin to the dialysis bath. This is still one of the most controversial aspects of your job as a dialysis technician. Heparin is a drug and every state has strict laws governing who may give prescription medications. However, many of these laws were written before the dialysis technician existed. Therefore, whether or not a dialysis technician is permitted to handle drugs of this type is often the decision and responsibility of the individual employer. Your dialysis unit, as do many throughout the country, allows technicians to give these medications.

Throughout the rest of his dialysis treatment you will be carefully monitoring your patient. Mr. Klopp is now very familiar with the possible complications of dialysis treatment. He will alert you if he experiences any problems. Also, the machine itself has a number of alarms and safety devices which will immediately warn you if a problem occurs between your periodic patient checks.

You leave Mr. Klopp to monitor another patient whose dialysis is already in progress. Mrs. Longley is a new patient in the dialysis unit. Both she and her family are still adjusting to her illness. Her kidney disease came, as it does for many people, as a complete surprise. She had experienced no unusual symptoms, but when she went to see her doctor for a routine physical, he found that her blood pressure was very high. An appointment was made with a kidney specialist, Dr. DeOreo, who made several additional tests and ordered a kidney biopsy. (A biopsy is surgical removal of a very small piece of tissue for microscopic examination.) The biospy confirmed the diagnosis of glomerulonephritis, a disease which is an inflammation of the kidneys. By the time of her second examination Mrs. Longley had already lost about 50% of her kidney function. She was immediately put on a strict diet and special medications were prescribed. However, as the doctor explained then, this treatment would not cure her. Eventually she would need dialysis or an organ transplant. Just five months later the rest of her kidney function was gone, and she began dialysis treatment at your Center.

Since coming to the Center, she has been doing reasonably well. She recently switched her hours to the evening so she can do her housework during the day and go to school part-time. Her husband watches their little girl in the evening while she comes for treatment. You check her blood pressure and pulse and carefully check the machine's settings. Everything appears normal. You ask her how she feels. She says she is a little cold and her muscles are beginning to ache. This may mean nothing or it could possibly mean an infection is starting somewhere in her body. You take her temperature. It is slightly elevated. Her symptoms now definitely point in the direction of an infection. You carefully notate her records and then personally notify the nurse-in-charge.

You return to check Mr. Klopp. So far, no problems, he reports. Everything is fine. You check the machine and monitor his vital signs. Yes, your own observations confirm everything is indeed fine. He then goes back to working on his stock statements. He uses dialysis time as extra work time.

The other patient you are monitoring tonight is also absorbed in his work. Tom Neale is a bright high school student who is planning to go to college next year.

One thing this young patient possesses is determination. He has already had one kidney tranplant. But, as sometimes happens with a donor kidney, Tom's body rejected the kidney about twelve months after it was transplanted. He is on dialysis again now, waiting for a new kidney, and is hopeful that next time his kidney transplant will take.

As you are monitoring him, you become involved in deep conversation. Tom wants a little advice about a girl he has been seeing. Like most teenagers, he doesn't want to talk to his parents about this. You're his confidant. While you are telling him how you see the situation, Mr. Klopp shouts from across the room. You hurry over to find out what the problem is.

He reports that he is feeling faint. Since he is an old-timer, he knows what this means. His body's blood pressure is dropping, and he is experiencing hypotension. You carefully check the machine. There is a tiny blood leak. It's quickly corrected. You then administer a saline solution to your patient, which helps restore normal blood pressure. Then you go back to Tom and his problem.

The rest of the evening goes without any other major difficulties. Mrs. Longley is doing fine. The nurse, on a doctor's standing prescription, administered an antibiotic to check her infection. Between you and Tom, his love life problem is solved, and Mr. Klopp manages to get you into a lively discussion about the Dow Jones averages.

As each patient finishes dialysis treatment, you again check their vital signs, remove the needles, and carefully swab and bandage their arms. Then you carefully disassemble all the equipment, and clean and sterilize it for the patient who will use the machine tomorrow.

It is just after midnight when you head home. But you haven't left the job completely. You think about your advice to Tom and wonder just how well he'll make out with his girlfriend. Two days from now you'll be back together and you will have your answer.

PERSONAL QUALIFICATIONS AND WORKING CONDITIONS

It is not hard to guess what personal qualifications a technician needs if you can imagine yourself as a dialysis patient. What would you look for in a technician who assists you? You would probably want a technician who:

- has an ability to work well under stress, and who can respond immediately to the many dialysis emergencies which might arise;

- has good powers of observation and is alert to subtle changes in the patient or machine which can signal trouble;

- is extremely attentive to detail, thereby preventing man made errors in dialysis treatment;

- has good mechanical ability and manual dexterity for preparing the patient and setting up the machine;

- has good communications skills to maintain patient records and work with patients, families, and professional members of the dialysis team;

- has personal sensitivity and warmth, and who can provide the psychological support patients need.

If this is the type of technician that you would want to care for you, you are beginning to understand what dialysis is all about.

The physical work environment is similar to any hospital or clinic. The psychological environment is unique. In one sense it is like a nursing home. Most patients are not going to get well, but life must go on to the fullest extent possible. It is also similar to working with seriously ill cancer patients, whose lives may be prolonged by treatment, but for whom a cure is unlikely. Death, despite excellent dialysis care, also is a very real fact of life in the dialysis unit.

Like any health professionals who work with sick patients, technicians are exposed to illness in varying degrees. In the case of the dialysis staff, exposure to hepatitis presents the greatest risk. However, good sterile techniques practiced by the technicians and all members of the dialysis team eliminate this as a serious job hazard.

Work hours vary with each employer. Technicians working with hospitalized patients may have to work a rotating evening shift or be "on call" for nighttime or emergency work.

Outpatient facilities operate differently. They usually follow a standard schedule that is convenient for patients. Generally, this means hours similar to a regular workday. Many centers are also open on evenings and weekends so patients can dialyze without interrupting work or family routine.

This job normally does not involve any unusual physical demands. With the exception of the very ill hospitalized patients, generally no lifting or positioning of the patients is required. The equipment is also mobile. While the setting up of the dialysis machine does require manual dexterity, it does not require physical strength.

DIALYSIS TRAINING

You may be surprised to learn that despite the complexities of dialysis care, the training for this profession is almost exclusively on the job (OJT).

As of 1978, Malcolm X College in Chicago offered the only degree program in the country specifically in nephrology technology. Many other colleges have had renal programs in the past, but because of the high operating expenses and other problems, they are no longer in existence. Several new programs currently are in the planning stages. The program at Malcolm X is here to stay. It has been in operation since 1968 and is the model for future programs.

Ohio State University offers a baccalaureate degree in circulation technology, which includes dialysis as a portion of its critical training. (See Circulation Technologist.)

The Malcolm X program is competitive. Thirty students are admitted annually. A high school diploma or equivalent with a minimum "C" average is the primary prerequisite for admission into the program. High school courses in the sciences are very helpful. Before the renal educational program begins, the student must take college courses in basic college math, chemistry, general biology, anatomy, and physiology. The renal technology program includes liberal arts and technical courses and extensive clinical training. For two semesters, students spend three days a week from 8:00 A.M. till 12:30 P.M. working in a dialysis setting under supervision. Upon the program's completion, students receive an associate college degree in renal technology. Because these graduates have a formal education, their job opportunities are excellent.

On-the-job training is a different picture. OJT programs vary tremendously. Their length and content are determined largely by the employer. Generally, OJT will combine classroom and clinical work experience. Basic patient care practices, principles of dialysis therapy, and elementary human anatomy and physiology with special emphasis on the kidney and kidney abnormalities are taught. The trainee also learns the basics of sterile techniques and emergency procedures including cardiopulmonary resuscitation.

Technician trainees in an outpatient dialysis setting, where the less complicated patient cases are usually seen, generally require three to six months of *closely* supervised OJT. An inpatient hospital unit, where acutely ill patients are treated, requires longer training, usually a minimum of one year.

Each employer determines the specific job requirements needed to qualify for a trainee position. In general, a high school diploma is the minimum educational requirement. Some college, particularly in the biological sciences, is desirable. Persons who have had prior working experience with patients, such as licensed practical nurses, nurse's aides, or ex-military corpsmen, may also be given preference. Employers also look for trainees who have emotional maturity, since dialysis is an emotionally demanding profession.

Trainee positions are seldom advertised in newspapers. Most persons become trainees by contacting employers directly; in addition to an employment application, a personal interview is required. Applicants may also have to submit evidence of their high school and college work, if any. Several employment references and a pre-employment physical are generally required as well.

PROFESSIONAL CREDENTIALS

A license is not required to work in this field. Though the duties for dialysis technicians vary across the country, there has been some progress in initiating basic standards in this profession. A national certification exam has been established, which sets standards for and tests the technician's minimum knowledge of dialysis principles and practices. In order to take the examination given by the Board of Nephrology Examiners, Nursing and Technology, a technician must be a high school graduate or equivalent, provide documentation of basic training, have one year of clinical dialysis experience, and submit appropriate letters of recommendation from his or her dialysis supervisor. Technicians who successfully complete the written multiple choice exam can proudly wear the initials CDT, Certified Dialysis Technician, after their names.

Since almost all training is on-the-job, certification is obviously not required for beginning employment in the field. But for the technician who wishes to remain in and grow with the dialysis field, this credential is very important. Technicians who want to change jobs or to advance to more responsible positions usually find certification is an important step to new employment opportunities.

JOB OPPORTUNITIES

Are there job opportunities in dialysis? Yes and no. There is really no clear-cut answer, since this profession is still emerging, still taking shape. There are many variables which must be considered when looking at the technician's employment future.

First, who will get the dialysis jobs? This decision is up to the medical directors of the individual dialysis facilities. As mentioned earlier, in some dialysis units RNs and technicians may have almost identical duties and work side by side with a supervising RN in charge. In other units, particularly a pediatric or hospital unit where more complicated dialysis patients are seen, the majority of those employees may be RNs, with few, if any, technicians on staff. However, in some dialysis units technicians may perform all the dialysis treatment, again under the supervision of a nephrology nurse.

On a pure cost basis, technicians have an advantage. They cost less—generally about 20% less than a registered nurse. Starting salaries vary with the geographic location and the particular employer. Generally, though, they fall into the $9,000 to $10,000 range—not a bad starting salary for someone who has trained on the job and has had to make no financial investment in training.

But employer dollars are only part of the picture. Federal dollars are also a major factor in employment outlook. Currently the government subsidizes 80%

of all dialysis care in this country. If this continues, and thus far there is no reason to believe it will not, the job opportunities for technicians should remain good to excellent.

More dialysis centers are needed. Even though there are currently about 785 dialysis facilities throughout the country, many patients still must travel several hours to reach a dialysis center. With continuing government support, more dialysis centers will probably be built to help correct this problem.

Home dialysis, where patients dialyze in their own homes assisted only by family members, is another alternative to this problem. Theoretically this would not only compensate for the lack of a nearby dialysis facility but, if all patients dialyzed at home, it could eliminate the need for outpatient dialysis facilities— and technicians—altogether. An extra advantage is the low cost of home dialysis care. It costs approximately $90 a day for home care, versus an average of $150 per day at an outpatient facility.

Though the government is supporting home care, it has not really changed the picture for dialysis care throughout the country. Many patients simply cannot dialyze at home. A family member may not be available to assist; the patient may be afraid or unwilling to assume the responsibility for his or her own care; limited space at home may make dialysis care impractical.

Another important factor that would seriously affect the job market would be a decrease in the number of patients requiring dialysis care. This, however, is unlikely. The number of patients requiring care has been increasing each year and this trend probably will continue.

Kidney disease is a much more serious problem than previously thought. Revised estimates indicate that some 13 million persons, rather than the 8 million previously recorded, suffer from kidney and urinary disease. Each person without proper treatment could become a future dialysis patient.

Several other factors are contributing to the increase in dialysis patients. Sophisticated diagnostic procedures are discovering kidney and urinary problems earlier. Our population itself is growing and, through better medical care, living longer. For example, about 2½ million people suffer from serious diabetes. Years ago, persons with this problem would die from the disease itself long before other complications, such as kidney disease, would develop. Today these patients have normal life spans as a result of good medical care. Many eventually will live long enough to develop end stage renal disease.

Until kidney disease can be prevented or cured, the number of patients needing dialysis treatment will never truly decrease. Realistically, this breakthrough will not happen in the foreseeable future. And again federal funding plays an important role.

In 1977 the government spent a little over $2 million a day for dialysis treatment through the Medicare program, but spent only $100,000 a day on kidney research. With this level of federal research support it is not likely that kidney disease will be conquered.

Kidney transplantation, the only "cure" for end stage renal disease, can't solve the problem either. Not every patient is a good candidate for transplantation, and for those who are, there simply are not enough kidneys to go around. Renal physicians estimate that in 1977 about 11,000 of the 36,000 dialysis patients were eligible for transplantation, yet kidneys were available for only 4,450 patients. Those lucky enough to receive a kidney still can't be considered cured, since there is always the danger of kidney rejection.

Though all the factors discussed thus far point to a very favorable employment outlook, you may be surprised to learn that employment turnover rate in the dialysis field is high.*

This happens chiefly because many persons enter dialysis without an adequate knowledge of what the job really involves. The appeal of on-the-job training, a good employment outlook, and reasonable wages motivate them to become technicians. Later they discover, by working, that they are not suited for the stress and psychological demands of the job.

Another contributing factor is the lack of clearcut advancement opportunities within the field. With most health careers, professionals have the opportunity to advance to supervisory, teaching, administrative, or other more responsible positions as they gain more work experience and/or education. Along with the greater job responsibility comes more pay and usually a change of job title. For example, the staff nurses become head nurses. These lines of promotion are fairly definite and are recognized by employers across the country.

As a dialysis technician no such promotion routes have been established. For dialysis technicians, employer practices largely determine what advancement, if any, is possible within a dialysis facility or unit. In some centers no real opportunities exist. Technicians who are experienced may "advance" in a sense by assuming the dialysis care for more complicated patient cases. But this advancement generally carries no new job title or increased pay. All supervisory or other advanced positions are reserved for the registered nephrology nurse. Technicians do, of course, receive periodic pay increases, but these are based on general seniority and/or cost of living.

In other centers there are some advanced positions for which technicians can qualify. For example, some facilities may divide the nursing care portion of dialysis from the technical part of dialysis treatment. The "chief technician" rather than a head nurse will supervise all technical aspects of dialysis treatment performed in the unit. This frees the head nurse to concentrate time and effort on the other patient aspects of dialysis care. In some dialysis facilities, the administrative work of the unit is separated from the nurse's role and taken over by a unit manager, who may be a dialysis technician.

While both these positions are open to dialysis technicians, moving into these

---

* This situation is not unique to dialysis treatment or to the dialysis technician. The employment turnover rate for all health professionals who work with critically ill patients is generally higher than average.

jobs almost always requires additional training at the college level. For the chief technician, additional course work in biological sciences—particularly physiology —would be important, in order to have a firm grasp on the technical part of the treatment. To qualify for the unit manager's job, the technician would have to take courses in administrative management.

Graduates of the Malcolm X program are notable exceptions. They are well prepared for advancement positions, since they already have received a formal education. Many of their first jobs are in complex care units, and within a few years of graduation many have moved into supervising or administrative positions. Their education also uniquely qualifies them for research positions.

Industry also offers opportunities for advancement. Technicians may be hired for sales or research positions, but again, additional college work may be necessary or highly desirable to be considered for these jobs.

Finally, technicians who want to remain within dialysis and yet advance, and who are willing to invest time and money in additional training, have another important option that they can consider: nursing. It is possible to earn a degree in nursing in as little as two years after high school, and some technicians do just that. After training they return as nephrology nurses, where their experience as dialysis technicians will serve them well.

HOW ONE TECHNICIAN SEES IT

If the work can be depressing, if the job opportunities seem uncertain, why would someone choose this profession? For many reasons. But one technician said it best. "When I got out of high school I didn't know what I wanted to do. So, I went to college and dropped out after a year. I still didn't know what I wanted to do. Then I got involved in dialysis. Now I know where I want to be. I am going to school again, part time, so I can do a better job. Eventually, when I have my degree, I know there will be job opportunities. As for the work, I find it motivating—a real turn-on, because as depressing as it can be, that is how rewarding it is too.

"I like my patients and sharing feelings with them. Surprisingly, they have a good sense of humor too. This job has changed the way I look at life. I can go home every night and get away from it. My patients can't. So I guess somebody has to be there to help. Why not me?"

For additional career information, write:

American Association of Nephrology Nurses and Technicians
2 Talcott Road, Suite 8
Park Ridge, IL 60068

For information on professional credentials, write:

> Board of Nephrology Examiners (Nursing and Technology)
> Middle City Station
> P.O. Box 15844
> Philadelphia, PA 19103

To give the gift of life through a kidney donation, write:

> National Kidney Foundation
> 2 Park Avenue South
> New York, NY 10016

CHAPTER XI

Between Here and Eternity

"Pump please."

"You're on."

This brief dialog sets the stage for the drama of human experience and medical expertise which are the hallmarks of open heart surgery. Inside a hospital a wife waits anxiously for news of her husband; inside the operating room her husband's life hangs in the balance, wholly dependent upon God, the surgeon's skill, and the marvels of biomedical technology. During the operation the patient's heart will be totally stopped. While he lies between here and eternity, a heart-lung machine will maintain the thread of life.

The machine itself is fairly simple, but the body functions for which it substitutes are extremely complex. This is no simple plug-in, hook-up piece of medical apparatus. Its operation requires the skill, knowledge, and expertise of a master physiologist. This special health professional is the perfusionist, a little-known but vitally important member of the open heart surgical team.

Though the surgeon generally receives all the credit for this operation's success, the perfusionist is virtually indispensable to that success. The perfusionist scrupulously monitors the patient during heart surgery and operates the heart-lung machine so that the patient's most basic body function—oxygen circulation to the body tissues—is maintained at the best possible level. Achieving this is no mean feat. It requires a special kind of technical precision equal to the skill of the surgeon's knife. As you understand more about perfusion you will begin to see why.

PERFUSION IN MEDICINE TODAY

Perfusion technology has expanded rapidly since the first open heart surgery took place in 1953.

By today's standards those first perfusions were fairly primitive. In those early days, most perfusion was performed by physicians. The technology was such that the physician's primary concern was simply oxygenating and pumping blood in order to maintain immediate life support. This aspect of perfusion, of course, remains unchanged today, but the explosion of knowledge of human physiology and improved technology now permits the perfusionist to concentrate on the quality of

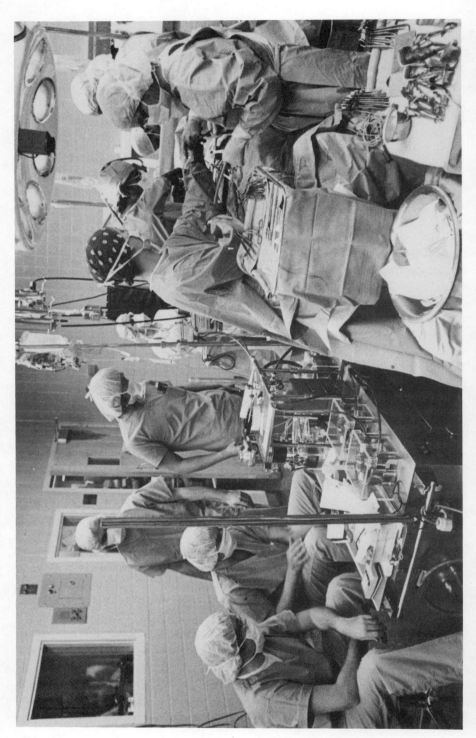

The open heart surgical team prepares for action. Note the heart-lung machine and team of perfusionists on the left. Courtesy of author's friend.

life as well. The perfusionist is concerned not only with what happens during surgery and immediately after, but with the long term physical and mental effects of perfusion on the patient.

Open heart surgery is not the only medical application for perfusion technology. Its use in organ transplantation is essential. Perfusion can keep kidneys or certain other vital organs alive—even outside the donor's body—for varying periods of time until recipients for the organs become available. Long term perfusion, lasting several days to two weeks, may aid some victims of severe chest trauma, such as a crushed chest or other major lung problems. Perfusion in this case allows the lungs to recover partially until they can resume major life support again.

This use for perfusion is not widespread; it still must be greatly improved and refined. Yet it does hold promise for the future. In fact, the greatest advances in this biomedical technology will probably be in the next ten to fifteen years.

THE BASICS OF PERFUSION TECHNOLOGY

During open heart surgery, the heart must be stopped so that defects and diseases of the heart and/or its major blood vessels can be repaired, replaced, or otherwise corrected. When the heart stops beating, a chain reaction occurs: the lungs stop as well. Oxygen does not enter the body; waste products, such as carbon dioxide, do not leave. Blood is no longer pumped through the body. Oxygen, which is fed by the lungs and carried by your blood stream, no longer reaches your body tissues.

Without life-giving oxygen these tissues begin to die, some sooner than others. Brain cells are particularly susceptible. Unless they are constantly fed with oxygen, brain damage occurs within brief minutes, and in less than ten minutes death results. Through perfusion, the body cells remain oxygen-nourished and cell damage is prevented.

Like dialysis, perfusion is a form of extracorporeal technology, meaning circulation outside the body. During perfusion the patient's blood supply leaves the body via a catheter (tube) which has been inserted into a major blood vessel of the heart. The tube connects the patient to the heart-lung machine. What happens once the blood reaches the heart-lung machine depends on the specific equipment being used. In a "bubble" oxygenator, the blood enters a chamber of the machine which contains fluid or donor-matched blood. Here, oxygen is bubbled through the chamber and blood, oxygen, and carbon dioxide are mixed. Carbon dioxide is eliminated and the newly oxygenated blood is pumped back to the patient.

A "membrane" oxygenator more closely resembles a dialysis machine. Upon entering the machine, the blood circulates through an extremely fine material which acts as a semi-permeable membrane. This material is much finer than that used in dialysis machines. It has to be, as it must transfer and transport gases in the blood, rather than chemical substances as in dialysis.

Inside the machine a two-way gas exchange occurs. Through diffusion, excess carbon dioxide (CO_2), a waste product, is removed from the patient's blood, and oxygen is introduced. Once this two-way exchange has occurred, the machine pumps the newly oxygenated blood back to the patient under great pressure. There, it circulates throughout the body, again feeding and nourishing body tissues. This membrane oxygenator mimics the natural process which occurs in the alveoli of the lungs. But it is far less efficient. Our lungs can oxygenate up to forty liters of blood per minute, while the machine can only handle about seven.

But despite the limitations, during perfusion the body's own heart and lung functions can be successfully replaced or "bypassed" by the machine. Consequently the procedure is commonly referred to as cardiopulmonary (heart-lung) bypass—bypass for short.

Bypass, in a nutshell, is a perfusionist's major responsibility. While this may seem simple in theory, in practice it is not. It requires the highest degree of discretion, judgment, and personal responsibility.

THE PERFUSIONIST'S ROLE AND RESPONSIBILITIES

The patient plus the machine sum up the perfusionist's major duties. The two literally function as one during cardiopulmonary bypass. Each patient and each bypass procedure is unique. As in all surgery, little can be considered routine or standardized.

The perfusionist's role with the machine begins with the selection, in consultation with the surgeon, of particular equipment for the bypass procedure. It must be specifically suited to the individual patient and type of surgery which will be performed. This selection process can be more involved than just deciding upon a particular machine. It may require the perfusionist to design a special system for the operation by adapting or modifying existing equipment on hand.

Before equipment can be used it must be properly set up, tested, and in top working order. A machine malfunction could be fatal to the patient.

Contact with the patient usually starts in the OR while the team is still prepping the patient. The patient's specific physiological needs for oxygen and other chemicals must be calculated. A grown man will require more oxygen to sustain his life than will a newborn infant. Individual body chemistry varies too, so the perfusionist must draw a blood sample to obtain a chemical profile of the patient. Once the patient's needs have been computed, the bypass machine must be adjusted so that the blood that will be oxygenated and returned to the patient matches, as closely as possible, the blood chemistry of the patient when his or her own heart and lungs are working.

But all this is just a starting point. Human physiology is never static. Even though the machine is adjusted once, throughout the operation it must be constantly readjusted to meet the patient's changing physiological needs.

So, from the beginning of the operation until its end, the perfusionist is actively involved—continuously monitoring both patient and machine, holding steady the thread of life so that the surgeon can mend the damaged heart.

Achieving good perfusion requires the skills of a technical artist, the knowledge of a scientist, and the decision-making ability of a field general. The responsibility that the perfusionist assumes is tremendous. If the surgeon does a great job, and the perfusionist does not, the patient is in trouble.

As a technical artist, the perfusionist must skillfully juggle many complex factors in order to maintain the patient's delicate physiological balance. Just as our own oxygen needs change with our activities (for example, we need more oxygen while we are working than while we are sleeping), surgery itself places unusual demands on the patient's body. Despite the fact that a patient remains motionless throughout open heart surgery, it is a physically gruelling experience. The body is subjected to great stress over a long period, sometimes six to seven hours. Any drug given to the patient also changes the body's oxygen demands. Sedation given before and anesthesia administered during the operation both alter the patient's physiological equation. Generally, patients receive other medications during surgery as well. In order to perform bypass itself, heparin or other anticoagulants are necessary to prevent dangerous blood clots from forming.

Administering anesthesia and other drugs, particularly heparin, often becomes a challenging responsibility for the perfusionist. Though administering drugs is still considered controversial by some, the fact remains that often the best way to administer anesthesia quickly and efficiently is via the heart/lung machine. Drugs needed to maintain near-normal physiology are given this way for the same reason.

Though a physician prescribes these drugs, he or she does so usually in the most general sense. The perfusionist generally works from a "standing" list of available drugs which the physician has prescribed in advance for use as needed during surgery. However, it is the perfusionist who must decide which drug is needed when, and in what dosage.

Why is this important responsibility left to the perfusionist and not the physician? For the simple reason that, from the standards of good patient care, there is usually little choice. Performing the intricate surgical heart procedures requires the surgeon's total concentration. Monitoring the patient for even the most subtle changes is another separate and full-time job. Changes, when observed, must be countered immediately by the perfusionist, using whatever appropriate drugs or machine adjustments are necessary. This requires that the perfusionist make independent decisions. In the OR seconds count. There is no time to discuss with the physician which drugs should be selected, and the necessary dosage.

But perfusionists do more than just react to problems; they must be able to anticipate them, and prevent them if possible, or at least to minimize them. To do this, extensive scientific knowledge is required. Not just physiology, pharmacology (the science of drugs), hematology (study of blood), and biochemistry, but an understanding of the surgical procedures themselves is required. Whatever the surgeon does at a particular time can have an impact on bypass, so the perfusionist must synchronize the two activities. Bioengineering principles are also involved. No machine can be depended upon to work independently without error or interruption. But in perfusion there is no room for machine malfunction. Consequently, the perfusionist must know how to make on-the-spot repairs and understand the limitations, hazards, and safety features of each and every piece of equipment used in extracorporeal circulation.

Finally, perfusion requires constant decision-making. The technologist must quickly recognize and instantaneously react to correct the countless problems which can develop with extracorporeal circulation, whether they be problems related to the patient's condition, to the surgical operation, or to the equipment itself. These problems are not infrequent occurrences; they can happen at any time, and do. Whatever decisions the perfusionist makes directly affect the patient. Should more oxygen be given? Is the carbon dioxide concentration too high? Does the patient need more fluids? These and countless other questions must be answered instantaneously, and decisions for appropriate action must be made.

WORKING ON THE TEAM

Bypass entails more than just working with the patient and carefully manipulating human physiology via the heart/lung machine. The perfusionist, as an integral member of the open heart surgical team, must work with other team members as well—particularly the anesthesiologist, the MD who administers anesthesia to the patient during surgery. While the anesthesiologist maintains overall responsibility for any anesthesia given to the patient and its effects, this, as mentioned before, often involves the perfusionist, since anesthesia may be given via the heart/lung machine. But even when anesthesia is not administered this way, the perfusionist and anesthesiologist must work together. Each patient receiving anesthesia reacts differently to it, even when undergoing "normal" surgery, when cardiopulmonary bypass is not being used. Extracorporeal circulation, however, adds an extra dimension. Patients, who react individually to anesthesia, react differently still when anesthesia is being given via the heart/lung machine. Therefore, the anesthesiologist and perfusionist must communicate closely. The perfusionist, who is closely monitoring the patient's body functions at the most basic chemical level, will be the first professional to observe the patient's particular reaction to the anesthesia. If the perfusionist's monitoring shows the patient is picking up too much oxygen as a result of the anesthesia, the anesthesiologist must be immediately notified so the medication rate can be adjusted.

Because perfusion is such a highly complex procedure, ideally it is not performed alone. Often two—and in some cases three—perfusionists are teamed together under the leadership of one who acts as a primary perfusionist. The primary perfusionist is the key decision maker and is responsible for the overall perfusion. The assistant, or "first assist," supports the primary perfusionist in all activities, whether it be checking and reporting on the current stage of surgery, calculating dosage rates for physiological changes, or simply recording patient information.

This record keeping, as you might well imagine, is extremely important. Every medication and its dosage, every chemical test result, every equipment adjustment —in short, all information concerning any aspect of perfusion—must be carefully recorded. This information documents the perfusionist's every action, and the patient's status throughout the operation. From a legal standpoint, this information is essential; from the patient viewpoint, it is critical. In the event that anything goes wrong, the surgeon, the anesthesiologist, and the perfusionist will need this information to show them precisely what happened.

But the only way to really understand what happens during perfusion and surgery itself is to be there. So come inside the open heart surgical suite and step into the shoes of the perfusionist.

THE SURGICAL SUITE

You're up early this morning—before the sun. You must be at the hospital by 6:30 A.M. You are the primary perfusionist on this morning's case. As you get ready, you are not listening to the news and the world events; instead, your thoughts are on tiny Marcie Siegel and the human events which will unfold in the next few hours.

Your patient, just four months old, is scheduled for the most important event of her life: open heart surgery. Dr. Nahmie will be repairing her heart, which has a peculiar congenital (meaning at birth) defect which affects four separate areas of the heart. Without surgery her future is predictable: she has none. This operation is essential if she is to grow to adulthood.

Though the actual operation takes place today, your work began last night when you visited the pediatric unit to review Marcie's chart. You carefully noted her height and weight, and the results of her blood and electrolyte studies. This information was necessary to help you determine her basic physiological needs and help you select the proper equipment. You noticed that her hematocrit, the test which indicated the percentage of red blood cells present in the blood, was high. This told you that one area of her heart, though defective, was perhaps not as seriously impaired as it might be in similar instances of this kind of birth defect.

Your phone call to Dr. Nahmie confirmed this and together you discussed the plan for her operation and the equipment selection. Dr. Nahmie has decided that deep hypothermia will be necessary to operate on this small patient. All the while you were talking to Dr. Nahmie, you were developing in your mind a mental picture of the equipment and its setup for today's operation. Advance preparation in perfusion is always important.

When you arrive at the hospital you quickly change into surgical garb: a surgical cap which completely covers your head and special surgical "booties" that fit over your shoes. These booties are specially made to insure electrical safety. Since the heart/lung machine, as well as other equipment used in the OR, is electrically operated, you must be grounded.

The patient and the OR technicians and nurses have yet to arrive. You quickly begin your basic equipment setup, assembling all nonsterile items first. You carefully check for electrical safety, machine leaks, and mechanical malfunctions, literally putting the machine through a dry run. Finally, when you are satisfied that the system is operating without a hitch, you leave to begin your scrub.

You will not be in the immediate area of the operating room field. Therefore, according to aseptic techniques, you are not required to do a full scrub, but your policy is to do one anyway. This is an added safety measure to help protect the patient against infection, which is the danger of any surgical procedure.

As another safety measure, your perfusion department practices "culturing": testing of both the patient's blood and fluids inside the heart/lung machine before and after the procedure. This can detect the presence of bacteria that can cause infection. If the cultures, which take several days to grow, are positive, then the source of the infection must be tracked down as soon as possible. Was the machine's fluid contaminated? Was it a break in aseptic technique on the part of the surgical team?

You are proud of your hospital's excellent record: less than 4% of all the cultures taken after open heart surgery in your OR are positive.

While you are scrubbing, your first assistant perfusionist, Ms. Fong, takes the necessary samples for culturing. Ten minutes later your scrub is through. You don a surgical mask and are ready to connect the sterile pieces of your equipment. Once it is assembled, you must carefully check the machine's operation again and recirculate fluid through the entire system. Now that the machine is completely operational, you can turn to other preparatory work that must be done.

You begin calculating Marcie's particular physiological needs. Using the height and weight measurement that you obtained last night, you calculate the exact surface area of her entire body. This will help you determine the proper circulatory rate for your patient. Because deep hypothermia will be used during the operation, her normal hematocrit will have to be altered. Blood, like other fluids, "thickens" with low temperatures. Therefore, her blood must be "thinned" so that it will flow easily through the tubing. The amount of fluid in the machine will have to be adjusted, as well as your dosage of heparin. You check to make sure all necessary pharmaceutical supplies, such as calcium, potassium, IV solutions, and Lasix and Mannitol—two necessary diuretics*—are on hand. Whole blood will be needed for the operation. Though it is the nurse's responsibility to make sure the blood is available, participants in open heart surgery work as a team and double-check each other. The blood has been brought to the OR. Each blood-donor slip must be carefully matched against each blood unit. There can be no mixups here. A mismatch could cause a serious reaction in your patient—even death. When the

* Diuretic: A drug which increases urine output.

blood has been checked, it can be added to the machine. You then double-check your hot and cold water lines, which you will need for cooling and rewarming the patient's body. Hypothermia requires a different oxygen and carbon dioxide level than does "typical" perfusion, so gas tanks must be carefully rechecked to make sure the proper combination is available.

Now little Marcie is brought into the room. The surgical procedure now begins. Open heart surgery of any kind is a delicate procedure, but when performed on such a tiny patient, it becomes even more complicated. Monitoring lines are being attached and inserted into her tiny body. These lines will monitor her arterial and venous blood pressure and the electrical activity of her heart—actually an EKG. Her life signals will be picked up, recorded, and then displayed on an oscilloscope screen, much like a TV. Throughout surgery you will carefully watch these pictures, which will give you valuable information on her well-being. Additional monitoring lines are attached to record her left atrial and pulmonary pressures.

Once monitoring lines have been set up, you draw a blood sample by siphoning off blood from the monitoring line. Though you reviewed Marcie's hematocrit and blood studies last night, this blood sample will determine precisely those same factors now, at the time of surgery. Her Activated Clotting Time must also be calculated. You must know how her body reacts before heparin, the anticoagulant, is introduced into her bloodstream. You perform the hematocrit and the ACT yourself, using the mini-lab that is a standard feature in the open heart operating room suite. The blood gas study that you need is more complex. It is sent down by messenger to the hospital pulmonary department for immediate analysis.

Within five minutes you have the results of all your tests and are able to make your final calculations. Once these are established, you can adjust your control settings and put the blood into the machine, and recirculate it to make sure it is properly mixed.

Ms. Fong has been watching the progress of the surgery and giving you intermittent reports on the surgeon's progress. "Her chest is open," she reports. Dr. Nahmie is inserting a special cannula into her heart vessels which will soon hook Marcie to the machine.

"Okay," he says. "We are going on bypass." Those words trigger you into immediate action. It is now time to connect the patient to the machine. Your sterile tube is ready but you cannot pass it manually to the surgeon. This could contaminate the tube and threaten your patient with bacterial infection. Each hospital has a special method for solving this problem. Yours uses a special mechanical device designed by the perfusion staff which allows you to pass the tube to the surgeon without using your hands.

Dr. Nahmie takes the tube. You notify Dr. DuBois, the anesthesiologist, of the heparin dosage you have calculated for the patient. He then adds the drug to her IV line. You do another ACT. Now that heparin is in her body, the clotting time will be dramatically different. Meanwhile, Ms. Fong thoroughly checks the equipment setup again, making sure that the line is properly connected. There can be no margin for error here. If the hookup is not perfect, the patient's life is on the line. "Okay," she says. "Okay, all hooked up," you report to Dr. Nahmie. "Can you please test?" he says. You again test the system. "The system is Go," you report. "Are you ready to go on bypass?" You listen attentively for his answer. There can be no mistaking the surgeon's reply. He must fully acknowledge that you are ready to proceed; then he himself must give you the go-ahead. "Go on bypass," he states. "You're on pump," you reply.

Initially you are on partial bypass only. Marcie's tiny heart is doing part of the work and the machine is doing the other half. You begin to carefully adjust the temperature controls, since the bypass machine will now be used to induce hypothermia. Using the machine, her body will be cooled from its normal 98.6 down to 65 degrees Fahrenheit. All the time you are bringing her body temperature down, you are carefully watching the many oscilloscope screens, watching her heart action, noting her blood pressure, checking her pulmonary function. Finally, you reach the desired temperature. You notify the surgeon: "You're ready for total bypass." Once again everything must be checked. "Okay, we are ready," you report. Dr. Nahmie acknowledges your statement. Total bypass begins.

Now it is you—the perfusionist—and the surgeon working together. You are both holding Marcie's life in your hands. While the surgeon repairs her anatomy, you maintain her physiology.

As the operation progresses, your concentration remains unbroken. You constantly sample Marcie's blood. With Ms. Fong's assistance, you perform hematocrit and ACT readings, send blood samples to the lab for electrolyte and blood gas studies, monitor her temperature control, and make sure that her arterial and venous blood pressures are maintained.

You and Ms. Fong work closely as a team, with you in charge. She assists you by making the calculations you request, and meticulously records all patient information. She also acts as a runner, watching the progress of the surgery and giving you bulletins. Using this information, you adjust the gas mixture and carefully control its flow. Hypothermia alters the anesthesia required for the operation, and you and Dr. DuBois must be in close communication.

Ms. Fong notifies you that Dr. Nahmie is ready for the second phase of the operation. He will stop Marcie's heart. In this particular case, bypass will stop too. Surgery on such a tiny patient requires the surgeon to operate in a completely bloodless area, or "dry field," so that all of the structures can be easily seen and repaired. This requires not only that the heart be stopped, but that all circulation must cease. This is possible with hypothermia. With the lowering of Marcie's body temperature, her oxygen demand dramatically drops. Therefore, her heart and circulation can be halted for the next two hours while the surgeon repairs her damaged heart.

Though you are not performing bypass during this time, you continue to monitor your patient. Ms. Fong announces that Dr. Nahmie is almost finished with the necessary repairs. You will soon be returning to bypass. Again the dialog is repeated. "Are you ready to go on bypass?" Dr. Nahmie asks. You again carefully test all of your systems. "Ready to go," you reply. "Pump, please," he says. "You're on." Though the dialog is brief, it is vitally important. You and the surgeon must coordinate your activities, with his direction, down to the moment.

You now start the rewarming process, bringing Marcie's body temperature gradually up to the normal level. This requires great technical expertise. You want to rewarm Marcie's body at the same rate that you cooled it. You also want to make sure that at every degree of temperature change, her oxygen levels are being maintained. Fluctuations in oxygen and carbon dioxide levels here are a sign of poor technique. They could also retard your patient's recovery following surgery.

Everything goes beautifully. In addition to checking blood pressure and hematocrit and other factors, you check the operation of the left ventriculator vent of your machine. You must make sure this pump is operating properly; otherwise blood will accumulate in and distend the left ventricular area of her heart, possibly causing permanent damage. Again, all goes uneventfully. Soon you will be off bypass altogether.

Ms. Fong reports that the surgeon is almost through. Just a few minutes more and the machine will have done its job. Suddenly an alarm goes off. You have just a split-second to decide what has happened. It's the arterial line. It's become disconnected. The oscilliscope shows a tremendous drop in Marcie's blood pressure. You have less than 15 seconds to remedy the situation. Now all your practice of emergency procedures must be put into action. You must work quickly. There is almost no time for thinking; you act almost instinctively. You quickly shut down the arterial pump and close off the venous return; at the same time, you clamp off the faulty arterial line so that no air enters the patient. Then you reconnect the arterial line. Before you can return to bypass, you must remove the residual air in the line. If it were repumped into the patient, the results would be fatal.

You tell Dr. Nahmie it is okay to go back to bypass. He gives the go-ahead, and bypass begins once more. Now, in addition to your other monitoring, you and Ms. Fong must find out what caused the accident and then correct the problem. Though today's emergency was not a common occurrence, in perfusion you must always be prepared for the unusual—whether it is a similar machine malfunction, or an unusual situation that the patient or the surgery itself presents.

The rest of the operation goes uneventfully. Dr. Nahmie announces he is ready to come off bypass. You respond and slowly start the bypass weaning process. Little Marcie's heart gradually begins to pump on its own, supported by the machine. As the minutes slip by, her heart takes up more of the work while the machine's role gradually diminishes.

Dr. Nahmie announces, "Now it is time to come off." "Okay," you reply. "We are off." Though bypass is officially over, your job is not completed yet. The machine is now used not to circulate the patient's blood, but to transfuse additional whole units into the patient. Dr. Nahmie has already specified the number of cc's that will be needed. Meanwhile, Ms. Fong is taking another sample for the final blood studies and culture on the patient. Her hematocrit is a little low, she reports. You notify Dr. Nahmie and recommend that additional blood be added. You also check Marcie's urine output. If it is not good, this means fluids will be building up in her body, making her heart work harder. Sure enough, it is a little low. She will need a diuretic.

Today's case is finally over. Marcie is being wheeled to the intensive care recovery unit, where she will be watched by a specially trained nursing team for the next several hours. The operation appears to be a complete success, but only the next few hours will tell for sure.

You carefully disassemble all your equipment, readying it for another case.

Nothing else is scheduled for today—that is, unless there is an emergency. But emergencies, it seems, never happen during the day. Just three days ago you were awakened at 2 A.M. by a hospital emergency call. Like a fireman, you had to respond immediately. Within minutes you were out the door—your third emergency this month.

You head for the dressing room to change back into your civilian clothes. You glance at the clock. It is hard to believe that almost five hours have passed since you first stepped into the operating room. You ditch your booties and soiled clothing into the laundry bin. Then you pin your small transistorized "call" device to your pocket. You wear your caller both inside and outside the hospital. Wherever you go, the hospital can page you by simply dialing your core number, 136003. After lunch you will spend the rest of the afternoon in the research lab. You will be testing an oxygenator that is being considered for purchase. But your thoughts keep drifting back to Marcie. Before going home, you will stop by the recovery room to see how your patient is doing. Your involvement with the case never really stops at the OR. You make it a point to visit all your patients following surgery. You are interested in more than just sustaining life during the procedure; you care about the quality of life afterwards.

PERSONAL QUALIFICATIONS AND WORKING CONDITIONS

Now that you have a better understanding of what perfusion is all about, you can well imagine that this is not a career for everyone. Perfusion requires a unique blend of personal characteristics, some which are shared with other health professionals involved in technology today:

- Good manual dexterity and coordination (needed to set up and operate the heart/lung equipment).

- An ability to make rapid and accurate calculations.

- An ability to organize, analyze, and coordinate information (needed for interpreting and applying the patient's medical data to cardiopulmonary bypass).

• An ability to work well under stress (essential for functioning in the open heart surgical setting).

But beyond these basic characteristics, a perfusionist needs other qualities. The perfusionist must be able to work well not just under stress, but under periods of continued stress. This is the normal work climate of the workday. Therefore, emotional stability is a necessity. While many health professionals must be able to organize, analyze, and coordinate information, the perfusionist must be able to do this quickly and to react immediately to any given situation. Time in the open heart surgical suite is measured not in minutes, but in seconds. Finally, innovation and an ability to make independent decisions are absolutely essential. Since the course of any operation is unpredictable, the perfusionist must constantly be creative in adapting to whatever situation may arise. He or she must be able to make the necessary independent decisions, and accept the responsibility which accompanies them.

This profession is undoubtedly one of the most demanding. While the job makes no unusual physical demands, the psychological climate is unique. The mental concentration needed by the perfusionist can become physically exhausting.

The work week in perfusion is not limited to 40 hours. It depends on the operating schedule. The perfusionist is also frequently on call for emergencies. In this profession, the words "on call" take on extra meaning. Because perfusion is such a highly specialized profession, hospitals who employ perfusionists usually have an extremely small perfusion staff. Consequently, when the perfusionist is on call, he or she shares this responsibility with but a handful of other perfusionists. Understandably, then, the chances of being called to the hospital to handle an emergency case are high. Throughout the course of this career you can expect to be called in the middle of the night, on holiday, and while relaxing at home or partying with friends. In short, this career, like that of the open heart surgeon, is a 24-hour-a-day job and requires a person with a strong sense of personal dedication.

PREPARING FOR TRAINING

Whether a perfusion program requires a high school diploma or some college for admission, the key to preparing for professional training is the same: a good background in science and math. This is absolutely essential for mastering the complex physiology involved in perfusion and for handling the computation necessary to perform cardiopulmonary bypass. Biology, chemistry, and math are the fundamentals. The perfusionist will work with the metric system of measuring, algebraic equations, percentages, logarithms, and exponents, and will apply knowledge of the gas laws, periodic tables, and states of matter. Perfusion requires more than just a working knowledge in these areas. You must be able to use these skills with ease and accuracy, under pressure.

PROFESSIONAL TRAINING

Professional training in perfusion is rigorous. In the past most training has been available almost solely on the job. This, however, is no longer true. Formal professional education is an absolute necessity.

Training is offered by hospitals, medical centers, colleges, and universities nationwide. Entrance requirements vary; some programs stipulate a high school education as the minimum requirement, while others demand at least one to two years of college with a strong science background. In addition, some programs require or give preference to students who have prior experience in a health field such as respiratory therapy, medical technology, operating room technology, or nursing.

Competition for training is stiff. The number of programs available are few; only ten accredited programs were in operation in 1978. Also, class sizes are generally small—approximately three to ten students per class. Because of these limitations, programs attract application from top-notch students. Despite minimum entrance requirements, many students who apply already hold college degrees.

Training programs last one to two years and include study of anatomy and physiology, pharmacology, perfusion technology, and surgical techniques. In addition, college programs include liberal arts and science courses.

Extensive clinical experience is an integral part of the education process. By graduation, each student must have performed a minimum of 50 clinical perfusions for which he or she had the primary responsibility. Some programs give the students an opportunity to learn techniques in other related areas. Ohio State University's Circulation Technology*, for example, covers dialysis and other applications of extracorporeal technology.

The Texas Heart Institute, professional home of famed open heart surgeon Dr. Denton Cooley, provides an opportunity for study in cardiac catheterization and research, among other areas.

At the present time, the American Board of Cardiovascular Perfusion accredits educational programs in the field. In the future it is expected that the AMA's Committee on Allied Health Education and Accreditation (CAHEA) will become the accrediting body in collaboration with other health profession organizations involved in perfusion.

Depending on the program, students receive a certificate or an associate or bachelor's degree upon completion.

Programs available, thus far, are evenly divided between universities and hospitals. Hospital programs are definitely less expensive. They may charge little or no tuition, and in some cases offer a stipend. University programs, on the other

---

* This unique program prepares students to function in many areas: dialysis, perfusion, cardiac catheterization, research, biomedical engineering, intensive and coronary care monitoring, delivery of cancer fighting drugs to the circulatory system, and other areas which involve the body's circulatory system.

hand, must charge tuition rates equal to that of other programs offered by the university. It is expected that in the years ahead the importance of an academic degree will increase. Students who complete academic programs will have greater opportunities for advancement in teaching, research, and administrative positions within the field. Ohio State University's Circulation Technology program has already proven this fact. Starting salaries for their graduates are higher than the national average ($12,000) for a beginning perfusionist. Within a few years of graduation, many have already obtained leadership positions within perfusion and other related fields.

PROFESSIONAL CREDENTIALS

The letters CCP are important initials after any perfusionist's name. They stand for Certified Clinical Perfusionist, indicating that the perfusionist has undergone a rigorous examination process administered by the American Board of Cardiovascular Perfusion.

This certification process is perhaps one of the most exacting of all health profession tests. To be eligible to sit for this certification exam, the perfusionist must be a graduate of an *accredited* training program. In addition, the perfusionist must have extensive clinical experience as specified by the American Board of Cardiovascular Perfusion. This takes into account not only the length of the perfusion experience, but its quality as well. The perfusionist must have performed a specified minimum number of independent clinical perfusions, meaning he or she must have acted as the primary perfusionist on the surgical case. Those eligible may complete a written and oral examination which tests, in depth, every aspect of the perfusionist's knowledge. Upon successful completion of the examination, the perfusionist is permitted to use the designation CCP: Certified Clinical Perfusionist.

Because perfusion is advancing so rapidly, certification is not given for a lifetime. The perfusionist must submit evidence of continuing education and clinical experience, which is acceptable to the Board, in order to prove continued competency in the field.

Though certification is not required for all initial employment opportunities, today it is an increasingly important credential for overall employment and advancement within the field. At the present time, perfusionists are not licensed in any state, and certification is used by many employers in lieu of a state license. Thus, employers selecting a CCP are assured of hiring a health professional who meets high standards.

JOB OPPORTUNITIES

As in all new technological professions, the job opportunity picture for perfusionists is multifaceted. Many separate factors may influence the job market in the years ahead.

On the positive side, there has been an annual increase in the number of open heart procedures performed throughout the United States, creating an increased demand for perfusion services. Surgical procedures themselves continue to improve, making previously difficult heart cases now treatable through surgical intervention. The public's growing awareness of certain surgical procedures, such as coronary bypass, the most widely performed open heart procedure, has contributed to increased surgical demand.

While these factors paint a rosy picture, there is another side, too. The profession is currently enmeshed in problems affecting all areas of medicine and allied health today: namely, medical malpractice and increasing federal regulation. Though the surgeon maintains ultimate responsibility for everything that happens within the OR surgical suite, in medical malpractice cases involving open heart surgery, anyone and everyone from the hospital administrator to the perfusionist may be included in a lawsuit.

In the area of federal regulations, the government has proposed a "non-reimbursement" policy whereby hospitals which perform fewer than 200 open heart procedures annually would no longer be eligible for compensation for their services through Medicare, Medicaid, Blue Cross, or Blue Shield insurance plans. This policy would affect 40 to 50% of the hospitals where open heart procedures are being performed today. Without reimbursement from private or public sources, most smaller hospitals that operate within this category will no longer be able to continue an open heart program. Fewer programs mean fewer perfusionists, and a potential employment surplus. However, it is possible that even if this policy is implemented, larger medical institutions will increase their open heart services to handle cases from defunct programs. This would diminish the overall impact on employment that this regulation might otherwise have. Still, the regulation is not yet in effect. It is currently in the planning stages, and no one, neither the federal officials, hospital administrators, nor the perfusionists themselves, can predict what the outcome will be.

Throwing another question mark into the employment outlook is the coronary bypass itself. The controversy over this procedure is still raging in professional circles. Is it of proven benefit to the patient? Does it really prolong life? Thus far neither side has been able to present conclusive evidence. But the eventual outcome of this tug-of-war could affect the employment market, since coronary bypass is the most frequently performed open heart procedure today.

Perfusionists who work in the clinical end of the profession are employed by hospitals, surgeons, or professional health corporations. In all cases, however, they must work in a hospital setting, regardless of who employs them. Open heart surgery can be performed only in a fully equipped surgical unit. The professional health corporations referred to are actually groups of perfusionists who work together, as physicians do in their group practices. Anywhere from three to six perfusionists, or more, may work together professionally. Hospitals purchase their services for a set fee per case.

For their hard work and personal responsibility, perfusionists are reasonably compensated. Starting salaries average about $12,000 a year; however, those with degrees may start several thousand dollars higher. Just as physicians have a wide variation in their earning power, so do perfusionists. Those with advanced degrees and considerable experience may command appreciably higher salaries. Perfusionists working for private corporations, which basically operate as profit-making organizations, often earn whatever the market can command. In these instances it is possible for an experienced perfusionist to earn upwards of $40,000 annually, depending on the "practice." However, they must also share the cost of an office, medical malpractice insurance, and other overhead expenses.

Research, teaching, administration, and industry also offer employment opportunities.

THE INSIDE STORY

You have seen what happens inside the open heart suite and the vital role the perfusionist plays. But what goes on inside a perfusionist's head during the tense moments of surgery? Each perfusionist would tell a different story. One interviewed said, "It really is more than a job. It is a way of life. Whether I am in the hospital or not, I am really on call, so my job is always in the back of my mind. When I am in the OR, I don't think about anything except the patient. I do my best, my very best, but afterwards I always ask 'Have I done enough?' "

For additional information, write:

> American Society of Extracorporeal Technology
> Reston International Center
> 11800 Sunrise Valley Drive
> Reston, VA 22091

For information on professional credentials, write:

> American Board of Cardiovascular Perfusion
> Post Office Box 20345
> Houston, TX 77025

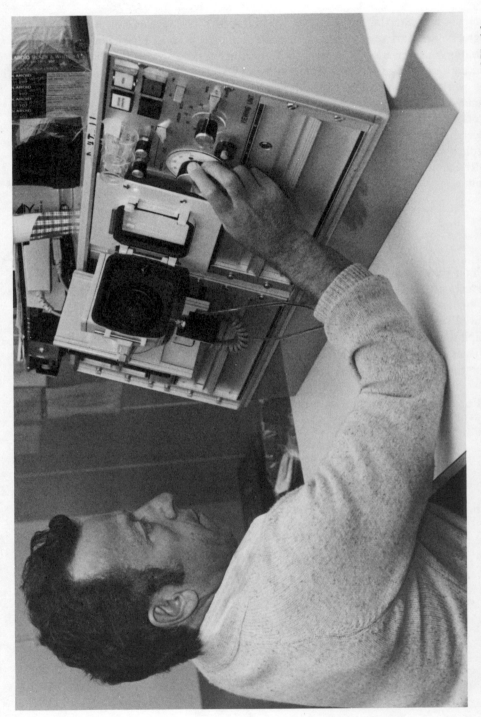

Biomedical equipment technician checks this CT scanner for proper functioning. Courtesy of National Institutes of Health.

CHAPTER XII

Medicine's Mechanics

Wherever you find electronic medical equipment—in the cardiology lab, the intensive care unit, the OR, or the emergency room—chances are you will find biomedical equipment technicians too. Just as physicians diagnose and treat health problems, and prevent them, biomedical equipment technicians handle problems of medical electronics—everything from emergency cases to routine equipment maintenance.

In just a short time this field has really taken off, developing from a simple repairman's job to a highly varied and important profession. Only twenty years ago a "modern" hospital had about ten pieces of electronic medical equipment; today it has over 2,000. And the number keeps growing with each new medical advance. Heart pacemakers, heart-lung machines, artificial kidney machines, blood pressure monitors, centrifuges, chemical analyzers, radiation meters, and spirometers are but a few of the electronic marvels used in medicine today. Though most people don't realize it, the biomedical equipment technician (BMET) makes a vital contribution to our health care—behind the scenes—by keeping these devices in top working order.

THE BMET'S RESPONSIBILITIES

Professional responsibilities in this career are as varied as the equipment with which the BMET works. This job requires a jack-of-all-trades.

First and foremost, BMETs are masters at repair. But before equipment can be repaired, the specific problem must be identified. This requires a thorough knowledge of how each piece of equipment functions. Simple knowledge of how to operate the equipment is also essential. In trying to pinpoint machine malfunctions, technicians must often test the machine's capabilities by actually operating it themselves. But repair is just one aspect of the technician's responsibility. Machines which hospitals purchase or rent must also be installed, properly calibrated, and maintained as well.

Maintenance is particularly important. That old adage, "An ounce of prevention," holds true for biomedical equipment technicians. A problem that is caught early can prevent more serious repairs later. This saves the hospital money, too—

not just the cost of major repairs, but the dollars lost when expensive and medically valuable instruments are not operating. Patients' safety is another critical reason for regular equipment testing and maintenance. A faulty cardiac monitor in a coronary care unit, for example, could cost a patient's life.

The BMET's job is definitely a "hands on" experience. Equipment must be taken apart, cleaned, oiled, and reassembled. Electronic circuits must be tested. Simple replacement parts such as pins and screws have to be shaped by a lathe. Tubes, switches, transformers, resistors, condensers—these are all machine parts with which the BMET works daily.

But surprisingly, not all work is with machines. Paperwork is another important part of the BMET's job. Careful records must be kept of all machine repairs, maintenance checks, and expenses. This log, which the technician maintains, provides valuable information which is used for many different purposes. First there is the obvious reason: a log helps the technician make up and follow a regular maintenance schedule. But it is also a vital tool to insure that recommended safety standards are being met. The operation of each piece of equipment must be measured, recorded, and checked against existing standards.

Beyond these reasons, a log helps to evaluate the machine's overall performance over a period of time. A hospital administrator will think twice before purchasing new equipment from a manufacturer whose current equipment is constantly breaking down. Manufacturers themselves are interested in learning of any technical problems and encourage BMETs to share this information with them. Lost contracts mean lower profits in a highly competitive market. Manufacturers are also constantly improving and refining their equipment. To do this, they depend on feedback from the field.

More paperwork comes in the form of professional journals and manufacturers' literature. By reading these, BMETs keep on top of the latest developments in their field. This enables them to speak with authority when they are asked to recommend new equipment. It is also a good way to obtain other information related to their job, such as information on changing safety standards.

But if you think this profession is strictly machine work and paperwork, you are wrong. There is definitely a "people" side to this career as well.

THE PEOPLE PART

You can't divorce medical equipment from the people who must operate it daily; consequently, when any machine is used, there is bound to be human error. In fact, operator misuse is a major cause of equipment breakdown.

The other health professionals described in this book are not usually the offenders. Their professional education includes training in equipment basics. However, today many other health professionals, particularly doctors and nurses, are working with electronic medical equipment. Few receive special training in the use of these devices as part of their basic education. Usually this is picked up—or not—later on in the job. This is where the BMET plays a vital educational role. When new staff is hired, or new equipment is introduced to a hospital unit, the technician often briefs the staff on how to operate it properly and safely. Other important tips, such as how to spot common problems and simple machine maintenance, are also covered. But of course, staff contact is not limited to doctors and nurses. As mentioned earlier, wherever electronic equipment is used, BMETs may be needed. So they are in touch with professionals of all kinds—physical therapists, medical technologists, radiologic technologists, and many others.

There is still more people contact—with patients. Not all work with machines is done in isolation. Often repairs must be made on the spot, where equipment and patients are located. A technician who becomes upset over the sight of blood or critically ill patients is of limited value. When working around patients, communication skills are a must. Patients well enough to be aware of their surroundings want to know who the technician is and why he or she is there. A bedside manner thus becomes important for the BMET too.

Now that you have been introduced to the BMET's job, why not try it on for size? Spend a day as a biomedical equipment technician.

A TYPICAL WORK DAY

It is 8:00 A.M. when you check into the hospital maintenance department. Before you can even switch into your lab coat, the department secretary hands you an emergency order which has already come in. It is a request from a nursing unit for repair of a defibrillator. This machine is used during cardiac arrest to deliver high, controlled dosages of electricity to the patient. The defibrillator can shock a stopped heart into action.

You select the tools that you think will be necessary for this job and then head to the patient unit. The nurse in charge points out the equipment in question. After carefully evaluating it, you come across the problem. It's a rather simple one, a faulty connection in the wiring. You quickly solder the wire back in place and then return to the maintenance department.

On the way back, you stop at the chemistry lab and pick up a pump for a chemical analyzer. This machine, an autoanalyzer, can perform a standard battery of tests on a blood sample. Within minutes, this machine can give the physician a complete chemistry profile of the patient. Over 25 tests can be performed, which would take a technician several hours to complete by hand. The medical technologist in charge is anxious to have this machine repaired as soon as possible. When it is out of use, understandably, a considerable backlog of laboratory work develops. When you checked out the machine yesterday, you discovered that a terminal board in the pump was short-circuiting. Today, back at your workbench, you will fix the pump and also give it a routine maintenance check.

Back in the lab, you make the necessary repairs and then carefully clean and oil the equipment. Then you record your activities in the log book. Before returning the pump, you calibrate a radiation meter which the radiology department sent down yesterday. You also clean the meter, and finally verify its operation by allowing it to run. It's A-OK. You take both the pump and the meter and head for the two departments.

At the chemistry lab, the technologist asks you to check a spectrophotometer. This machine performs chemical analysis by measuring the transmission or absorption of light energy in blood or fluid samples. You can't discover any problems. It seems to be working correctly. You tell the technologist this and ask her to keep a careful watch on the equipment. You then carefully notate your log. You will want to re-evaluate this piece of equipment early next week.

A lab technician who is working in the corner of the room spots you and hurries over with another problem. A washing machine which washes glass equipment used in various laboratory tests has broken. Technically, this is not your department; this is a mechanical problem rather than an electrical one. The hospital machinist should handle this. But you know he is busy, so you volunteer to make the necessary repairs. After repairing the machine you head for the radiology department to deliver the radiation meter.

On the way back there is a stop at the intensive care unit. Two new staff members have been hired, neither of whom have worked in an ICU before. The intensive care unit is equipped with a great deal of sophisticated medical equipment, so your briefing for the two new staff members will be especially important. When you arrive the two nurses are already waiting. You spend the next half hour discussing the operation of the equipment, basic electronics, and operator and patient safety.

Nurse Curtis is particularly concerned about electrical safety. She has heard stories about hospital staff being electrocuted in the line of duty. You smile and tell her that you haven't lost a nurse yet. By following the basic safety rules you have outlined, she should have no problems. Helping rid hospital staff of any fears they may have about working with complex electronic instrumentation is an important part of your staff education process. You also explain to the nurses that you are on hand to answer any of their questions any time and to handle any problems as well. They are both grateful for this basic orientation. Understanding electronic equipment and its proper use makes their job easier.

It's almost lunch time. Today you are meeting the hospital engineer for lunch in the cafeteria so that you can discuss some new equipment which the hospital is considering purchasing. Informally, over a sandwich, you discuss the possibilities. The chemistry lab needs another new machine and the hospital engineer is interested in your recommendations. You have already checked your log book and are ready to suggest a particular model that you know has caused little trouble. You and the engineer discuss together what you know about this type of equipment in general and about this manufacturer in particular. You offer to obtain the manufacturer's sample sheets on various models before making an official recommendation. Since you are one of the three BMETs on the hospital staff, your recommendations are heavily relied on by medical staff when deciding about medical equipment purchases.

After lunch, you spend a few hours in the maintenance department at your workbench, repairing various devices. A safety alarm is out on a dialysis machine. An oxygenator is malfunctioning. A blood pressure monitor needs rewiring. As you are completing work on the monitor, you hear your name being called over the loudspeaker. You are being asked to report to the coronary care unit.

When you arrive, the nurse in charge explains that one of the cardiac monitors is on the blink. She leads you over to a patient's bedside. You take one look at the equipment and inwardly groan. It is a mess. Whoever hooked it up obviously did not know what to do. Your outward expression, however, remains unchanged. You can't convey your feelings to this patient. That would frighten an already sick person. The nurse leaves and you chat with Mr. Haas a bit. Rather than tell him that you are here to fix his machine, you explain that you are just going to give it a little tune-up. He complains that electricity from the machine has been giving him chest pains. You assure him gently that this machine does not give off electricity, but picks up the electrical activity of his heart. That puts him a little more at ease. Understandably, having all this electrical equipment around and attached to him is a strange experience.

The problem is soon corrected. You return to the maintenance department and find a request has come in to repair an electronic marker in the operating room. You are not even sure what an electronic marker is, but you report to the operating room without delay; you'll look at it anyway.

This is one aspect of your job which makes life interesting. There is always the unexpected—some new piece of equipment that is being introduced, or some new problem. Flexibility is really the key to your job. You always have to be ready to apply basic electronic principles to a new situation.

At the OR you are introduced to an electronic marker. It's similar to other devices you worked with, and with a bit of tinkering the problem is corrected. You mention to the operating room supervisor that all new electronic equipment that the department orders should be routed to you first. This helps you to do your job better. If equipment goes through you first, you can become familiar with it, order parts for support, and study the basic literature from the manufacturer on maintenance and repair. You jot down in your log the name of the manufacturer and the style model, and make a note to call the manufacturer in the morning so you can obtain all the necessary data on this machine. Next time there is a problem, you'll be ready.

You hurry back to the department to prepare for tomorrow. You finish logging in all the day's activities and then make up requisitions for new supplies and replacement parts. Tomorrow you will be out all morning. But though you won't be officially at the hospital, you will still be officially on the job. A manufacturer's convention is in town, and this will give you an opportunity to view and compare the latest equipment of over 100 different manufacturers. Finally, about an hour after your normal workday is over, you can call it a day.

Would you call this a satisfying workday? If so, perhaps this career is one that you should consider.

PERSONAL QUALIFICATIONS AND WORKING CONDITIONS

The biomedical equipment technician needs many and varied skills in order to perform this job:

- Manual and finger dexterity, good eye and hand coordination, and mechanical aptitude (needed to work with intricate pieces of equipment).

- Good observation and an eye for detail (needed for identifying problems and painstakingly correcting them).

- An ability to work under stress (BMETs often have to make emergency on-the-spot repairs).

- Good communications skills (needed for working with hospital staff, hospital administrators, and equipment manufacturers: the BMET should be able to explain the fundamentals of electronics and the basics of equipment clearly and simply).

- Good organizational ability (needed for organizing the workday, ordering supplies and replacement parts, and keeping schedules and other documentation as necessary).

Working conditions vary with the employer. In hospitals, the 40-hour work week may require working a rotating shift, weekends, holidays, or being on call for emergencies. During an emergency situation, the BMET must be prepared to work longer hours until the emergency is over.

When working for industry, the BMET's job may involve extensive travel to areas where the company's products have been installed in order to maintain or repair equipment. In these instances too, emergency situations may arise, causing abrupt changes in plans and unexpected or prolonged absences from home.

The physical demands of the job change with the workday. One "normal" workday may find the technician in many different departments of the hospital, while another "normal" workday may be spent entirely at the workbench. In general, there is little direct supervision, and the BMET must be prepared to assume a great deal of personal responsibility for organizing and performing his or her work.

PREPARING FOR TRAINING

If you are interested in mechanics, electronics, physics, and math, and do well in these courses, you may have an aptitude for this field. Courses in chemistry, biology, and physiology are helpful also, because as a BMET you must understand the relationship between the human body and the electronic principles. English and other courses which will build your communications skills are important educational assets. BMETs must work with patients, patient care staff, hospital engineers, and administrators, which requires the ability to communicate clearly.

PROFESSIONAL TRAINING

In the past, most BMETs learned their craft through on-the-job training and experience. With the increasing sophistication of medical devices and the increasing number of them on the market, this no longer holds true. Today most biomedical equipment technicians learn their profession through formal education programs in community colleges or technical institutes.

Currently, 32 such training programs exist in the United States. Some schools refer to their programs as medical electronics technology or biomedical engineering technology. Others still award degrees in electrical engineering, with special emphasis in biomedical instrumentation or biomedical electronics coursework. These programs generally last two years and award an associate arts degree.

During this educational program, students study anatomy and physiology, electronics, mathematics, biomedical instrumentation, chemistry, physics, basic liberal arts, and communications. Training also includes clinical work or field experience. This "hands on" experience may be provided in a school lab, but frequently it takes place at a hospital or other clinical facility where students work under the close supervision of an experienced BMET, a hospital or medical engineer. The student's training emphasizes not only general biomedical techniques, but also such specialty areas as radiology, nuclear medicine, and research instrumentation.

For students who are not college-minded, another training route exists—through the military. Both the Army and the Air Force offer one year of concentrated training programs in biomedical technology for military personnel. These BMET programs are rated among the best of all available programs, including college programs.

Costs of college training will vary. Community colleges generally charge little or no tuition. Private colleges and technical institutes may charge higher tuition. The military training, of course, is free; however, students must fulfill a service obligation. Also, the military cannot guarantee in advance that you will be placed in a BMET program.

Those persons who already have excellent skills in electronic equipment repair, though not in biomedical equipment repair, may enter the field through equipment manufacturers. Some manufacturers have trainee programs for persons already experienced in electronic instrumentation. This training is also free, and during the traineeship the person receives a salary.

Admission requirements for BMET college programs are typical of those for any other college programs. Evidence of a high school diploma or equivalent, an entrance examination, and a personal interview may all be required. Competition for admissions varies throughout the country.

PROFESSIONAL CREDENTIALS

Because this field is still new, still changing and growing, no licensing or certification is presently needed for employment. However, the Association for the Advancement of Medical Instrumentation does maintain a certification program for biomedical equipment technicians. This provides the technician with an opportunity to be formally recognized as having demonstrated a general knowledge of the biomedical equipment field. In order to sit for the certification examination, a BMET must complete one of the following requirements: two years of work experience plus an associate degree in biomedical engineering technology or military training, or three years of work experience plus an associate degree in electronics, or four years of work experience in the biomedical field. In addition to the experience and educational requirements, professional employment references must be submitted. Upon successfully completing the examination, a technician is designated as CBET, certified biomedical equipment technician. As stated before, certification is not required for employment, but it definitely expands the BMET's job opportunities.

JOB OPPORTUNITIES

The employment scene for BMETs is good and growing. Not all opportunities are in hospitals. Many BMETs work for biomedical equipment manufacturers, medical supply houses, and contract maintenance companies. In industry, emphasis is on installing and repairing the company's medical equipment and training medical personnel in the proper use of this equipment.

Government, through the military service, veterans' hospitals, the U.S. Public Health Service, the National Research Institutes, and other governmental agencies, employs BMETs. The responsibilities are similar to those in "civilian" hospitals.

Some BMETs may act as individual contractors, servicing a group of small hospitals. By sharing the services of a BMET, a hospital that might not be able to afford a full-time technician can still receive the BMET's valuable and needed services.

It is expected that hospital employment for BMETs will increase in the years ahead. This is due not only to the increasing use of medical electronic devices in health care, but also to the growing realization on the part of hospitals that a BMET can save dollars through prevention and maintenance. Because this field is still so new, the job descriptions and salaries for BMETs vary. Entry-level BMETs, those who are new graduates of associate degree or military programs in biomedical technology or electronics, can expect to earn between $10,000 and $11,000.

In general, the new graduates can perform a variety of basic tasks, but usually work under supervision. As the BMET gains more experience and proficiency in working with the whole variety of medical instruments, supervision diminishes. The BMET is then often responsible for supervising other personnel as well as for department administration.

This field is changing rapidly. Each year new equipment is introduced. Therefore, advancement for BMETs is based heavily on experience and continuing education, which broaden and deepen the technician's capabilities. With this combination it is possible for the BMET to advance to the position of biomedical engineer, a health professional you will meet in the next chapter.

IT'S A GOOD LIFE

How do those people working in the field see it? As one technician said, "The field is a challenge. It keeps me on my toes. I have to constantly keep reading and learning and growing. I feel I am in touch with the latest in what is happening in medicine today. But the best part is that I really like what I do. During high school I always enjoyed taking apart and fixing any machine I could get my hands on, whether it was a car or a power mower. Now, as a BMET, I have turned my hobby into a full-time job. It's a nice way to make a living."

For additional information on the biomedical equipment technician and professional credentials, write:

Association for the Advancement of Medical Instrumentation
1901 Fort Myer Drive, Suite 602
Arlington, VA 22209

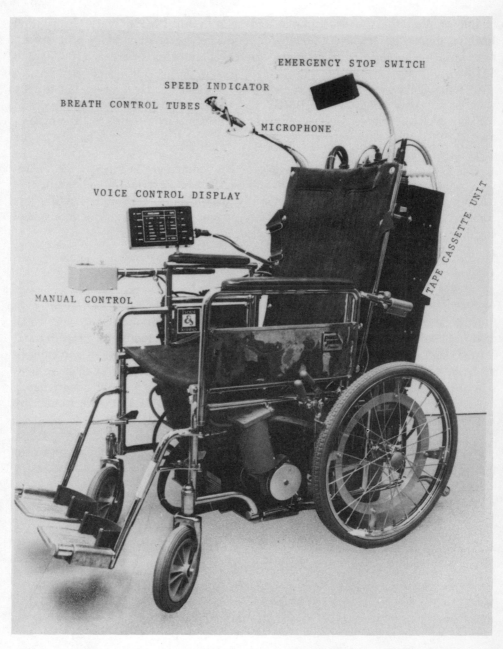

EMERGENCY STOP SWITCH

SPEED INDICATOR

BREATH CONTROL TUBES

MICROPHONE

VOICE CONTROL DISPLAY

TAPE CASSETTE UNIT

MANUAL CONTROL

Designed by biomedical engineers, this motorized wheelchair can be operated by a person totally paralyzed in both arms and legs, via voice command. Courtesy of New York University Medical Center, Institute of Rehabilitation Medicine.

CHAPTER XIII

From the Drawing Board

A 22-year-old man, permanently and totally paralyzed by an upper spinal cord injury two years ago, is now a freshman at a state university. He is able to use his hand and arm to print, type, and answer the phone, and he can now drink from a cup. Small accomplishments for an average person, but to this young man they are miraculous.

What made this miracle possible? A relatively new and unique science—biomedical engineering. In broadest terms, biomedical engineering is a science which applies the principles of engineering and technology to understanding and solving mysteries of biology and medicine. But within this definition lies a world of exciting technical possibilities for medicine and man.

Biomedical engineering and its professionals, biomedical engineers, have made substantial contributions to health care. As for public acclaim, biomedical engineers may themselves remain unsung, but their accomplishments have not gone unnoticed. Dialysis and heart/lung machines, electrocardiograph and EEG machines, linear accelerators, ventilators, heart pacemakers—almost every medical device you have read about has come into existence largely due to the important work of these health professionals.

And yet, developing sophisticated medical equipment is just one aspect of their role in health care today. The biomedical engineering field is vast. In addition to developing treatment and diagnostic equipment, artificial organs, and other medical devices such as cardiac pacemakers, engineering principles are applied to many other areas of health care. For example, biomedical engineering helps to:

- evaluate the effectiveness of drugs, prosthetic devices, and medical equipment;

- monitor patients via a computer system, whether patients be in intensive care units, coronary care units, or on a regular patient floor; monitor astronauts in space and divers under the sea;

- develop and utilize new energy sources, such as chemical or nuclear cells;

- develop systems for insuring electrical, mechanical, chemical, radiological, or nuclear safety;

- design information systems to keep medical records and diagnostic data from physical examination or laboratory testing.

These are but a few of the ways in which biomedical engineering contributes to the delivery of health care today. Biomedical engineers, in essence, take fundamental engineering principles, such as electronics, fluid dynamics, mechanics, optics, radiation, and thermodynamics and apply them directly to health and health-related areas.

For example, fluid dynamics, the science that deals with the forces exerted by fluids and their relationship to motion, can be applied to the various fluid systems of the body. The body contains many different kinds of pumping systems, which serve to help digest food, excrete wastes, and maintain the environment of cell tissue. Our bladder, for example, has been engineered so that it can accommodate an increasing volume of urine without increased internal pressure, until it is time for urine to be expelled. The uterus, which delivers newborn infants to the outside world via rhythmic contractions, is another pumping system. Biomedical engineers who are interested in fluid dynamics can concentrate their attention on the body's most obvious pumping system, our circulatory system. Currently underway is a project to develop an artificial heart that will keep that circulatory system in operation when the human heart fails.

As you can see, the possible applications of engineering to health are endless. Indeed, in biomedical engineering, we have only just begun.

WHAT'S IN A NAME?

Before delving any further into this field, let's set the record straight. Many different professional titles have been assigned the biomedical engineer, often creating confusion. Since the 1960's, the term "biomedical engineer" rather than "bioengineer" has gained recognition by the professional engineering organizations as the preferred occupational title for engineers working in biology and medicine.

But falling within the broad biomedical engineering area are several areas of specialization: bioengineers advance the understanding of biological rather than medical systems. Medical engineers are "development specialists" using engineering to design medical equipment or devices such as artificial organs and diagnostic and treatment machines. Clinical engineers, sometimes called hospital engineers, are "improvement" specialists, using engineering to improve (and maintain) all aspects of the delivery of health care—everything from insuring equipment safety to designing information systems for patients or health care employees. Bioenvironmental engineers are "protection" specialists, protecting our health and the quality of life, whether it be human, animal, marine, or plant life, by safeguarding our environment from toxic substances and pollutants.

But whatever they are called, these engineers by any other name remain biomedical engineers.

THE TEAM EFFORT

Biomedical engineers are a unique breed: part physician, part scientist, and all engineer. These are the special talents which they bring to the research team. Though the research field is often characterized as lonely, today research is seldom carried out alone. Increasingly it is a team effort, bringing together biomedical engineers, physicians, biochemists, physiologists, and other scientists from the medical, life, social, and physical sciences. Each member is equally important and dependent on the others in the research effort. The biomedical engineer contributes special engineering expertise, coupled with medical and biological knowledge to attack the problems at hand.

But the team isn't limited to those just named. Research technicians play an important supporting role in the research effort, providing extra hands to carry out basic tests and procedures. Still, the team is not complete. The patients can't be forgotten either. Though they are not team members in the official sense, the patients who participate in research make a significant contribution to medical advancements that will benefit us all.

PROFESSIONAL ACTIVITIES

What kind of work activities does the biomedical engineer encounter each day? This is difficult to predict. Much depends on the area in which the biomedical engineer specializes and the particular project at hand.

In biological, medical, and bioenvironmental areas, where the emphasis is strongly on research and development, the biomedical engineer may engage in a wide range of activities. Time may be spent working alone at the drawing board, drafting mathematic models or designs; meeting with other team members to collectively brainstorm or test ideas; programming a computer to test or develop theories; working in the laboratory, putting into action the ideas worked out on paper; working on a hospital floor with patients, putting into practice the products tested in the laboratory.

The research process is complex and requires careful following of scientific methods. This means long hours of trial and error, carefully testing and retesting each design or device before it can be used with patients. Research triumphs, when they occur, do not happen overnight. They are usually the result of years of work and dedication.

In clinical (hospital) engineering, the workday may be entirely different. While these engineers often engage in research, they may have additional job functions as well. Within a hospital or other health facility, they may investigate the cause of electrical accidents; modify medical equipment and systems; conduct staff seminars on personal and patient safety; recommend to hospital administrators new equipment purchases, after carefully researching the market. With much of their work they see immediate results. The description of the biomedical equipment technician's day in the previous chapter will give you a sense of what clinical engineering is about. Clinical engineers, however, have greater responsibility and are educated to perform more complex tasks. Their time is too valuable to spend on routine equipment repair.

For all biomedical engineers, writing and recordkeeping are important professional activities. Professional reports must be written and records must be meticulously kept, whether they deal with research itself or with hospital operations. Because every aspect of biomedical engineering is changing so rapidly, all engineers must keep abreast of the latest developments. Attending professional meetings and conferences, reading professional journals, and continuing education through seminars or special courses are required.

Because the professional activities of the biomedical engineer are so varied, it would be impossible to introduce you to a typical day, but in the next section, you will see a small sample of the exciting projects in which biomedical engineers are involved today. You, too, can participate in these or other projects should you decide this field is right for you.

In addition to all these activities, many biomedical engineers are responsible for supervising other employees, such as research or biomedical equipment technicians. Teaching or administrative duties may also be a part of their activities.

THE WIDE, WIDE WORLD OF THE BIOMEDICAL ENGINEER

The paralyzed young man mentioned earlier is not a character from a writer's imagination. He is a real person, one of fourteen spinal cord patients who are participating in a biomedical research project. These patients are testing one of the most promising experimental electrical devices engineered to date. The device uses an electrical system to compensate for and replace lost nerve and muscle function. It consists of a transducer, attached to his chest; a stimulator, placed under the wheelchair; and tiny stainless steel electrodes, about one-third as thick as a strand of hair, implanted in the hand muscle.

Even the implantation of these electrodes requires the application of engineering principles. Instead of surgery being used to implant the electrodes, the wires are coiled into a spring and placed inside a hypodermic syringe; just the tip of the wire extends beyond the needle's point. When the needle is inserted into the patient, the wire then catches in the muscle and is implanted.

By learning to move the shoulder muscles, which are usually left intact in an upper spinal cord injury, the young student can now initiate hand and arm movement himself. When he moves his shoulder muscle, the degree of movement is picked up by the transducer attached to his chest. The transducer then signals the stimulator, which in turn activates the implanted electrodes to produce muscle contractions, allowing him to grasp and move his hand.

Training the muscles is a hard and tedious step-by-step process. The biomedical engineer, in concert with physical therapists or other health professionals, has to train the patient to consciously direct the shoulder muscles. (You can see how difficult this is if you try to move an individual shoulder muscle without moving the entire shoulder.) Before this training process can even begin, sufficient muscle strength must be restored. Then the biomedical engineer must select the ideal electrodes for the patient after carefully noting his muscle responses to various electrical current levels.

But the system is still not perfect. For instance, electrodes can migrate within muscles, so physicians must make frequent checks to determine when electrodes are no longer exactly in place, and then remove them and insert new ones. Biomedical engineers are also working to improve the feedback system, so that eventually patients can determine the force of their grasp without having to observe their hands.

Now let's turn to the bioenvironmental engineering side of this field. Perhaps no greater tragedy exists than that of a malformed baby. When birth defects result from outside chemical or environmental factors which could have been prevented, the situation is even more tragic.

To prevent this situation from occurring, biomedical engineers at the National Institute of Environmental Science are developing models to study the different mechanisms which produce these birth defects. Various environmental agents and drugs are known to affect reproduction and development, but their specific molecular effects during the early stages of development are still not well understood. These scientists are using mouse tissue and organ culture systems to determine the potential effect of direct application of test agents. In the long run they hope to be able to predict birth defects, and to prevent them from occurring in human life.

In the clinical engineering arena, biomedical engineers are applying the same techniques they use in monitoring astronauts in outer space to monitor unborn infants in "inner space." This monitoring is performed in the hours shortly before the infant "astronaut's" entry into our own world. This development actually is an offshoot of the space program, where space engineers applied radiotelemetry, a radio relay system which permits communication with satellites in outer space. By applying this principle first to animal models and later to selected patients, the biomedical engineering team developed a fetal monitoring system whereby the unborn infant's heartbeat can be continuously detected and recorded.

This system provides physicians with important information. By checking the heart signals and the effects of labor on the infant, this information can tell the physician whether or not the infant is experiencing distress which could be harmful. Fetal monitoring is not necessarily used for all maternity patients, but for those high-risk mothers who have special pregnancy problems, this new technique is invaluable.

Though the technique has been available since 1970 and is widely used today by hospitals throughout the country, the biomedical engineering team is constantly

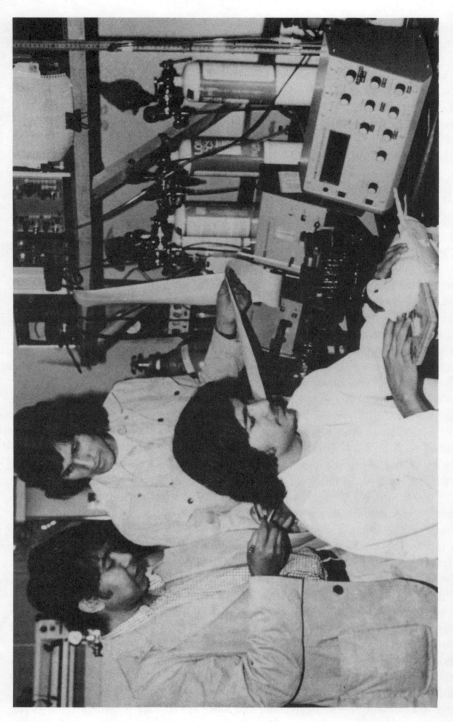

These students are studying the respiratory pattern of pigeons to understand how birds cope with flight at high altitudes without oxygen loss. This knowledge may be applied to developing special respiratory devices for patients. Courtesy of Division of Research Resources, National Institutes of Health.

searching for new ways to improve biomedical technology. The research team has already designed a refinement to this system. In the original system, the mother was virtually bedbound, attached to the machine by wires which severely restricted mobility. The new monitor permits the mother to move about freely in the often long hours before birth.

The new system uses microelectronics, the miniaturization of complex electronic circuits into small packages. By miniaturizing a radio transmitter circuit in much the same way that complicated clock circuits are miniaturized into a digital watch, the engineers were able to develop a tiny radio transmitter less than 5 cm. (two inches) long, complete with its own battery power supply. It is attached to the fetus by a scalp electrode. A telemetry receiver picks up the baby's heartbeat and displays it on an oscilliscope.

Then there is the radiopill, an innovative diagnostic invention of the biomedical engineer. This is a small sealed transmitter which, when swallowed by a patient, transmits physiological data such as temperature, pH level, or pressure within the patient's body to the physician. It is powered by a mercury battery and can be recovered and reused. The beauty of the radio pill is that it eliminates the need for more difficult, unpleasant diagnostic tests.

In the area of biomaterials, researchers are working on an electrode device which can be implanted in the inner ear, thereby opening up a world of sound to a formerly deaf person. Conventional hearing aids are of little or no value to the approximately 300,000 profoundly deaf persons in the world, but for the profoundly deaf person who still has partial nerve function, this implantable hearing aid could be the answer. The device would make use of the remaining nerve function and transmit electrical signals from the ear to the brain.

Results of experiments thus far with more than twenty deaf persons are encouraging. When a single electrode was implanted into the cochlea of the inner ear, loud sounds, such as a doorbell ringing, could be heard.

Perhaps the most controversial area of research today is genetic engineering, which has far-reaching importance and holds a potential for both good and bad.

A major breakthrough in genetic engineering came in May of 1974, when researchers found that they could combine the genes from an animal, the toad, with those of common bacteria. This was an unprecedented scientific feat. Ultimately "gene transplants" might be useful in producing bacteria capable of synthesizing valuable substances such as antibiotics or insulin, but they also hold potential for danger. A bacterial strain could accidentally be created which would be resistant to drugs or capable of producing substances harmful to man. When combining animal and bacterial genes, another possibility arises. Animal genes might carry instructions for making tumor viruses which can be easily attached to bacteria, thus possibly creating an increase in the risk of cancer.

Current research is still going on under the strictest control measures. Just where this area of research will lead, no one can predict.

The examples you have just read about are but a small slice of the biomedical engineering field. Research projects of all kinds are being carried out throughout the country, projects which can match every scientific interest.

If science engineering and medicine both interest you, perhaps a career as a biomedical engineer will interest you as well.

PERSONAL QUALIFICATIONS AND WORKING CONDITIONS

An aptitude for science, adaptability, and an analytical mind are the key qualifications for this field. Biomedical engineers must constantly analyze, organize, and coordinate information, and then apply it to medical and biological problem-solving. This is their life's work. Adaptability is also important in a field where each day may bring new changes.

Depending on the work assignments and the areas in which the engineer specializes, good manual dexterity and eye-hand coordination are often required. Communication skills are another must, since biomedical engineers must be able to communicate effectively both verbally and in writing. Information must be shared with the research team, physicians, patients, and other scientists world-wide.

Overall working conditions are largely determined by each employer, but in general they are good. A clinical engineer's hours are usually dictated by hospital policy. Generally, this requires working a daytime shift as well as being on call frequently to handle special problems as they arise. However, in a research setting the picture may be different. Although research laboratories may follow a regular 9-to-5 schedule, often work schedules are flexible and can be made to suit your own hours. However, this seldom means a less than 40-hour work week—in fact, the opposite is true. Most researchers put in extra time, whether it be by staying late, getting in early, or working weekends.

PREPARING FOR TRAINING

Science and math, and plenty of both, are the basic elements of educational preparation for the biomedical engineering field. At the high school level a good preparatory curriculum might include: 2 years of biology, 1 year of chemistry, 3 to 4 years of mathematics, 1 year of physics, 4 years of English, and 3 years of history, social studies, or other electives. A foreign language, particularly French, German, or Russian, can be helpful too, since many important scientific journals are published in these languages. Beyond this, communications courses, particularly those which build reading and writing skills, are essential. Biomedical engineers who cannot communicate effectively are of little value in a scientific community.

For high school students, the Junior Engineering Technical Society (JETS) offers a unique opportunity to test interest and aptitudes in biomedical engineering.

The program, which is designed for junior and senior high school students, is similar to 4-H or Junior Achievement programs and is sponsored by major engineering societies and leading employers of engineers. Among the programs which JETS offers its members are industrial tours, speakers, social events, and science competitions. Though schools usually sponsor local JETS chapters, students can also join the program as individuals.

In JETS the emphasis is on all aspects of engineering, not solely on biomedical engineering. But, since a good biomedical engineer must first be an excellent engineer, it is a good way to explore interest in this field.

Among JETS' specialized programs are the National Engineering and Aptitude Search and the Self Directed Search. The former is an aptitude test that helps students find out whether or not they have verbal, numerical, science, and mechanical abilities, all essential for engineering success. The Self Directed Search is a test which the students take themselves. It identifies occupations of particular interest to them. JETS also sponsors a special summer studies program for post-11th-grade students. For a two-week period during the summer, students are exposed to mathematics, physics, and engineeering subjects on a university engineering campus.

Another program, MITE (Minority Introduction to Engineering), an offshoot of JETS, encourages minority students to consider engineering. The program is now sponsored by the Engineers' Council for Professional Development. More information on the JETS and MITE is available from the organizations directly, which are listed at the end of this chapter.

PROFESSIONAL TRAINING

Be prepared for intensive education, combining engineering and science courses such as electronics, heat and mass transfer, mechanics, materials, calculus, thermodynamics, and computer technology with biological and medical studies such as anatomy and physiology, organic chemistry, biophysics, medicine, pharmacology, and psychology. Courses in medical terminology, basic English, and technical writing are frequently included in the curriculum.

In the past, education specifically in biomedical engineering was available only on the masters and doctoral (Ph.D.) level. Now, in addition to those programs, there are over 100 undergraduate programs in biomedical engineering. Bachelor programs take four years to complete, masters usually two, and Ph.D.s take three to five years after college.

Whether programs are on a bachelor's, master's, or Ph.D. level, tremendous variety exists. Unlike other professions about which you have read, there is no single basic curriculum which must be followed to prepare for this field. Consequently, programs vary from those offering a specific degree in biomedical engineering to those offering a general engineering degree in electrical, mechanical, civil, or chemical engineering with an option or concentration in the biomedical field. Other schools offer just a few basic biomedical engineering courses.

Selecting a program, then, should be done with great care. Each curriculum should be analyzed, and you should know in advance the objectives of the program. Is it oriented to hospital engineering or to research? Does it concentrate on biomedical instrumentation? Does it stress computer applications to biology and medicine?

In evaluating a program, keep in mind that first and foremost it should emphasize a strong engineering curriculum. Medical sciences, no matter how good, cannot be substituted for engineering basics. Rather, medical sciences should complement and support engineering studies. Why is this so important? Simply because as a biomedical engineer you will be depended upon by the research team for your *engineering* skills, which no other member of the research team can provide.

A key to evaluating a school's engineering excellence is whether or not it has been accredited by the Engineers' Council for Professional Development (ECPD), the accrediting body for all engineering programs nationwide. An ECPD-accredited program will offer a solid engineering background.

If you look briefly at some actual programs, you will begin to appreciate the diversity of education within the field.

Boston University's College of Engineering offers an undergraduate degree specifically in biomedical engineering. The program emphasizes biomedical electronics, computers in medicine, and mathematical models in biology and medicine, and is strongly oriented toward medicine. Fairleigh Dickinson University also offers a degree specifically in biomedical engineering, but without a standard curriculum. It tailors each academic plan to the student's background and research interests. Their program is sponsored, interestingly enough, by the College of Science and Engineering and the School of Dentistry. Among the research areas on which this program concentrates are prostheses (artificial devices which replace missing body parts), blood flowmeter, and data processing in hospital systems. Rice University in Texas offers such an option in biomedical engineering through its electrical, mechanical, or chemical engineering departments. Rice's program is research-oriented with a focus on cardiovascular-pulmonary areas, vision, neurophysiology, and biomechanics.

As you can see from this brief highlight, programs do vary a great deal. In addition to evaluating the engineering, medical, and biological curriculums of individual programs, you should also consider your particular interests. Many schools offer an "internship" or short-term work-study experience in a hospital, clinic, or other medical setting.

In general, programs are competitive, and usually only superior students are selected. At the masters and Ph.D. level, a student must usually have a good science and/or engineering undergraduate background before he or she will be admitted. Admissions procedures generally follow those of other college programs, including a transcript of all previous academic work, special entrance examinations, completion of a special application form, letters of recommendation, and, in some instances, a personal interview. Costs vary with each program, but generally overall education is expensive.

A recent trend has been the use of the undergraduate biomedical engineering degree as preparation for entrance into medical schools. While there are comparatively few biomedical engineering majors among the approximately 15,000 applicants to medical schools each year, their average acceptance rate is higher than that of students with traditional science backgrounds.

The undergraduate biomedical engineering degree should not be considered an end point. Full professional development within the field requires a masters or doctoral degree. Because at the present time so few undergraduate biomedical engineers are in the job market, it is difficult to evaluate the full potential of the bachelor's degree in biomedical engineering.

PROFESSIONAL CREDENTIALS

All states require professional engineers, whether working specifically in biomedical engineering or not, to hold a state license. The license is usually administered after the successful completion of a special state examination. Graduation from a state-recognized program and work experience are required to sit for the exam.

In a few states, biomedical engineers are licensed separately when they are working within the clinical engineering specialization. In addition to licensure, certification is given to clinical engineers by two professional organizations, the Association for the Advancement of Medical Instrumentation and the American Board of Clinical Engineering. Hospitals located in states where licensing of clinical engineers is not mandatory often require certification for employment.

JOB OPPORTUNITIES

Employment opportunities in biomedical engineering look bright, especially for those with graduate degrees. The Department of Labor predicts that the employment of biomedical engineers is expected to grow faster than the average for all occupations through the mid-1980's. Many schools educating biomedical engineers report that they have had little difficulty in placing their graduates.

As previously mentioned, it is still too early to predict the effect of the bachelor's biomedical engineering degree. Experts continue to debate whether the health system will continue to absorb these graduates. Most employers agree that the reason some graduates cannot find employment in this field is that usually their education has prepared them for a strong role in neither engineering nor medicine and biology. The importance of a good engineering background in biomedical engineering cannot be overemphasized.

Employment opportunities are indeed varied. Biomedical engineers can be found working in hospitals (usually those containing 250 beds or more) large clinics, or medical centers. Industry offers a wide range of job possibilities. In the automotive and aerospace industry, biomedical engineers are working in such areas as the life sciences, safety, and anti-pollution. In the pharmaceutical industry, they can apply their talents to research, testing, and marketing new drugs or health products. Of course, within industry many opportunities exist related to research and development of new electronic or mechanical instruments, or synthetic substitutes for human body parts, from artificial kidneys to artificial blood vessels. Jobs are also available as sales representatives for these products.

Looking to government, the National Aeronautics and Space Administration (NASA) employs engineers, especially in their life sciences division. The Food and Drug Administration employs biomedical engineers to help establish standards, safety, and effectiveness of medical devices and drugs. In the Department of Health, Education, and Welfare, the U.S. Public Health Service and the National Institutes of Health are two major employers of biomedical engineering manpower. Finally, the Department of Defense and Department of Transportation use biomedical engineers in developing programs of highway safety and environmental and pollution control.

Universities and colleges also offer varied jobs for biomedical engineers, as either teachers or researchers or a combination of both.

Salaries depend on the employer. But generally salaries are good, especially at the graduate level. A beginning biomedical engineer at a bachelor's level can expect to earn between $13,000 and $15,000 a year. At a master's level one may earn between $15,000 and $18,000 a year. Graduates with a Ph.D. degree earn slightly more. With additional education and experience salaries can advance rapidly, especially in industry.

PROFESSIONAL PAYOFF

If you decide to become a biomedical engineer, you must expect many years of training, long hours of study, and the expenses of higher education, and you might well ask yourself, "Is it really worth it?" Walter Evans of Case Western Reserve University wondered too. Now he knows. "After studying for six years to earn a master's degree, my career choice is beginning to really pay off. Not just in dollars, though my salary is good, but where it really counts, in my everyday work. I am working on two different projects now. One, as part of a research team, and the other, a small project I started on my own. So every day something new is happening, there really isn't enough time to get everything done. Making science and engineering work, in the areas where it counts most, makes my job one I wouldn't trade for any other."

For additional information on biomedical engineering, write:

Alliance for Engineering in Medicine and Biology
4405 East-West Highway
Suite 404
Bethesda, MD 20014

Biomedical Engineering Society
Post Office Box 2399
Culver City, CA 90230

For information on professional credentials, write:

Association for the Advancement of Medical Instrumentation
1901 North Fort Meyers Drive, Suite 602
Arlington, VA 22209

For information on special programs, write:

JETS
United Engineering Center
345 East 47th Street
New York, NY 10017

MITE
Engineers' Council Professional Development
345 East 47th Street
New York, NY 10017

CHAPTER XIV

Which Career for You?

You've just met over a dozen health professionals, each different, each unique, but which career is right for you? Where should you put your time, energy, and talents?

You can't—and shouldn't—attempt to answer this question until you take three important steps:

1. Read even more about the careers in which you are interested.
2. Investigate those careers firsthand.
3. Carefully evaluate each. Decide how well each career matches your own particular interests, aptitudes, and career goals.

This simple three-step process will help you make the right decision. Each step is essential. No matter how informative any book may be, it is still just the beginning in your career exploration. Try these practical suggestions for tackling those three important steps.

STEP ONE

The professional health organizations listed for each career described in this book are additional sources of written information. But they are by no means the only sources. Almost every profession publishes a journal to keep its members on top of the latest developments and issues in their field. These professional journals are another excellent source of information. While much of the material you will find in the journal is highly technical, you will usually find articles devoted to career issues as well. National salary surveys, continuing education, changing state licensure or certification requirements, and new educational developments are just a few of the areas which are often discussed. A journal can also give you a preview of issues about which you, as a future member of the profession, should be concerned—whether it be malpractice, changing technological developments, or the latest research findings.

Another invaluable feature of most journals is the job opportunities or job wanted section. These listings can give you a national perspective on the job market scene: What salaries are being offered regionally by employers? What educational or other professional requirements are employers looking for? What specialties within the field are most in demand?

Professional associations and journals aside, the schools that can prepare you for your career are another major source of career information. Almost every school has a brochure or catalog which is available upon request. These not only outline specific admissions requirements for the program, but contain other important information as well. Educational costs and financial aid are just two areas of interest. But, in addition, most contain general career information.

When you have read more about the profession you are interested in, you are ready for step two, your own personal career investigation.

STEP TWO

Before you begin step two, have ready a list of practical questions which will give you more insight into the field. Keep in mind that whatever you have read about the career is still secondhand information. How you "size up" the career and your future is what really counts. A career may sound very exciting, but you must be aware of the day-to-day realities of doing any job. This is where career glamour fades.

The best source for firsthand investigation is experience, by working on a paid or volunteer basis in a health facility. Here you can observe health professionals in action. They can also share with you, in detail, information which can be only briefly touched on in this book. They can tell you what professional training is like, which schools they recommend, what they like and dislike about their job. What are their goals within the field? How much independence do they have on the job during the regular workday? Where do they think the field is going in the future?

If you talk to ten different health professionals you will probably get ten different perspectives on the career, but when you look at them together, as a whole, you will begin to find the answer to your career puzzle.

Getting a beginning-level paid job in the health field depends on many factors: whether you meet the minimum age requirements, your education and related work experience, and how you go about your job hunt. Part-time and summertime jobs can be particularly difficult to obtain, so if you are looking here, start your job hunt as soon as possible. The best time to contact potential employers is early— *before* you need that job.

The personnel directors of health facilities are the most obvious contact, but not the only ones. Often, contacting department supervisors directly can result in a job offer. Supervisors often know about possible openings in their area well ahead of the personnel department.

Hospitals shouldn't be your only focus in your search for employment. Try other health facilities as well, whether they be nursing homes, special clinics, or research or laboratory facilities.

Volunteer positions are a different story. Generally speaking, you should have little trouble in securing a volunteer position. Almost every institution needs and depends on volunteers.

Don't expect too much from a volunteer position. Volunteer work is based on the concept of providing supplementary and complementary services to patients and hospital staff. Volunteers never *substitute* for paid employees. What you will be permitted to do within the hospital or health facility depends largely on the policy of the individual institution. A large teaching hospital, where nurses, physicians, and other health professionals train and where research is conducted, may offer a greater variety of volunteer opportunities. However, this isn't a hard and fast rule. A small institution, where the volunteer director personally knows each volunteer, may be more open to developing a special volunteer spot tailor-made to your interests. No matter where you volunteer, let the volunteer director know what you hope to get out of your work. Volunteering is a two-way street. You are giving your time, and should receive something in return. But to make a good placement for you, the director needs this information.

Volunteering or paid work aside, there are other ways you can explore your career interests.

- Visit a hospital, laboratory, or other health facility where you, as a trained professional in that field, might work some day. Many institutions hold regular tours. The director of public relations or the chief administrator's office should be contacted to make the necessary arrangements.

- Visit health professions schools. Like health facilities, many schools hold open house days. Arrangements can usually be made through the Office of Admissions or by contacting the professor in charge of the program.

- Take courses related to your career interests. This is an excellent way to test your interest and ability in the science area. If you have been out of school for a while, even if you had science during high school or college, a refresher course will help you determine if you are ready to begin school again. In addition to science and math courses, why not take a course in cardiopulmonary resuscitation, sponsored by the American Red Cross or American Heart Association? You will not only test your interest in the health field, but at the same time you will learn skills that could save someone's life.

Once you have gotten all the facts and explored each career in depth, you are ready for the final step: self-evaluation.

STEP THREE: THE MOST IMPORTANT STEP

The key to career selection lies here, in your self-evaluation. Though interest and aptitude tests, career counseling, and advice from family and friends may all assist you in the process, ultimately, the buck stops here with you. Here are some simple suggestions to help you with your evaluation:

- Decide what you want from a career, and how much time and effort you are willing to invest to reach this goal. The salary, job market, the type and time of training required, and personal job satisfaction are all factors you should consider in making your career decision. But only you can decide *how important* each factor is in determining your final choice.

- Analyze the work activities and environment associated with each career. Does this job require working a great deal with your hands, with equipment, with people, with information, or with a combination of these? Will you work alone or as part of the team? Will you work frequently under pressure or stress? Will you be required to accept a great deal of personal responsibility? Then ask yourself if you now enjoy performing similar activities under similar circumstances. Your hobbies, clubs, school, work, or other activities you enjoy can help you answer this question.

- Analyze the skills and education needed to perform each job successfully. Is college or college-level training required? How important are science, math, and reading skills, manual dexterity or mechanical ability, an ability to analyze, organize, and coordinate information? Then ask, do my abilities *realistically* match those required? Your schoolwork, present and past, is one important clue, but if it doesn't measure up, your effort, not your ability, may be all that is lacking. One senior student in a hospital radiation therapy program had failed high school physics, a course generally considered an important prerequisite for the radiation therapy field. At the time he didn't think it was important. Now that he is in training, applying the knowledge of physics daily, he realizes its importance. Today he's at the head of his class. Of course, he was lucky enough to find a program which gave him a chance to prove he had the ability, though he hadn't used it. If this might be your problem too, start doing something about it now. Take a remedial or refresher course and start building those areas in which you are weak.

If you take the time to tackle steps 1, 2, and 3, you should make a career decision that is right for you. This isn't easy. It does take time, work, and effort, but it pays off where it counts the most . . . your future. After all, your career is where your future begins.

Professional Journals

These professional journals are published by the professional organizations that represent the careers.

Radiologic Technology	For Radiologic Technologists, Radiation Therapy Technologists, Nuclear Medicine Technologists
Journal of Nuclear Medicine	For Nuclear Medicine Technologists; published by the Society of Nuclear Medicine
Medical Ultrasound	For Diagnostic Medical Sonographers
Respiratory Care	For Respiratory Therapists and Respiratory Therapy Technicians
Analyzer	For Cardiopulmonary Technologists
American Journal of EEG Technology	For EEG Technologists and EEG Technicians
OR Tech	For Operating Room Technicians
AANT	For Dialysis Technicians
Journal of Extra-corporeal Technologists	For Perfusionists
Annals of Biomedical Engineering	For Biomedical Engineers and Biomedical Equipment Technicians

Educational Programs

**Electroencephalographic Technician/Technologist,
Nuclear Medicine Technologist, Operating Room Technician,
Radiation Therapy Technologist, Radiologic Technologist,
Respiratory Therapist, Respiratory Therapy Technician**

These programs represent the most current listing available as of this printing. Readers are advised to contact the professional organizations directly for more up-to-date information. Schools should be contacted directly for information on their programs. The author wishes to thank the professional organizations for their cooperation in providing these school lists.

SCHOOLS

Programs accredited by the Committee on Allied Health Education and Accreditation of the American Medical Association.

KEY:
Electroencephalographic Technician/Technologist	[1]
Nuclear Medicine Technologist	[2]
Operating Room Technician	[3]
Radiation Therapy Technologist	[4]
Radiologic Technologist	[5]
Respiratory Therapist	[6]
Respiratory Therapy Technician	[7]

ALABAMA

Birmingham
Carraway Methodist
Medical Center [5]
Jefferson State Junior
College [5]
University of Alabama in
Birmingham [1, 5, 6]
Veterans Administration
Hospital [2]

Gadsden
Gadsden State Junior
College [5]

Huntsville
Huntsville Hospital [5]

Mobile
Mobile Infirmary [5]
Providence Hospital [5]

Montgomery
Jackson Hospital &
Clinic [5]
St. Margaret's Hospital [5]

Tuscaloosa
Druid City Hospital [5]

Tuskegee
Veterans Administration
Hospital [5]

ARIZONA

Flagstaff
Northern Arizona
University [5]

Phoenix
Arizona College of
Medical, Dental and
Legal Careers [7]
Biosystems Institute [6, 7]
Good Samaritan Hospital
—Samaritan Health
Service [4]

Maricopa Technical
Community College
[3, 5]
St. Joseph's Hospital &
Medical Center [1, 7]

Scottsdale
Scottsdale Educational
Center, Inc. [7]

Tucson
Arizona College of
Medical and Dental
Careers [7]
Pima Community College
[5, 6]
St. Mary's Hospital and
Health Center [5]
Tucson Medical Center [6]
University of Arizona
Medical Center [4]

ARKANSAS

Fort Smith
Sparks Regional Medical
Center [5]
St. Edward Mercy Medical
Center [5]

Little Rock
Baptist Medical Center [5]
Little Rock V.A. Hospital
[7]
St. Vincent Infirmary [2, 5]
University of Arkansas
Medical Sciences
[2, 3, 5, 6]

CALIFORNIA

Alta Loma
Chaffey Community
College [5]

Aptos
Cabrillo College [5]

Bakersfield
Bakersfield Adult School
[3]
Bakersfield Community
College [5]

Berkeley
Institute of Medical
Studies [7]

Burbank
St. Joseph Medical Center
[4, 5]

Burlingame
Peninsula Hospital and
Medical Center [5]

City of Industry
La Puente Valley Adult
Schools [7]

Costa Mesa
Orange Coast College
[1, 5, 6]

Duarte
City of Hope Medical
Center [4, 5]

El Cajon
Grossmont Community
College [6]

Eureka
General Hospital [5]

Fresno
Fresno City College [5, 6]

Fullerton
Fullerton Community
College [5]

Hawthorne
Hawthorne Community
Hospital [5]

Inglewood
Daniel Freeman Memorial
Hospital [5]

Lancaster
Antelope Valley College
[5]

Loma Linda
Loma Linda University
[2, 4, 5, 6]

Long Beach
Long Beach City College
[5, 6]

Los Altos Hills
Foothill Community
College [4, 5, 6]

Los Angeles
Charles R. Drew
Postgraduate Medical
School [2]
Children's Hospital of Los
Angeles [5]
East Los Angeles College
[6]
Kaiser-Permanente
Hospital [4]
Los Angeles City College
[2, 5]
Los Angeles County—
USC Medical Center
[2, 4, 5]
Martin Luther King, Jr.
General Hospital [5]
UCLA Center for the
Health Sciences [4, 5]
Veterans Administration-
Wadsworth Hospital
Center [2, 5]
White Memorial Medical
Center [2]

Lynwood
St. Francis Hospital of
Lynwood [2, 5]

Martinez
Contra Costa Medical
Service [5]

Marysville
Yuba Community College
[5]

Merced
Merced College [5]

Modesto
Memorial Hospital of
Stanislaus County [2]

Napa
Napa College [6]

North Hollywood
Valley College of Medical
Dental Assistants [7]

Oakland
Meritt College [5]
Oakland Public Schools
[7]

Orange
St. Joseph Hospital [2]

Oroville
Butte Community College
[6]

Oxnard
St. John's Hospital [5]

Palmdale
Palmdale General Hospital
[2]

Palo Alto
Veterans Administration
Hospital [2]

Pasadena
Huntington Memorial
Hospital [5]
Pasadena City College [5]

Redwood City
Canada College [5]

Riverside
Radiation Therapy
Medical Group, Inc.
[2, 4]

Sacramento
American River College
[6]
Sacramento Medical
Center [2]
Sutter Community
Hospitals [2, 4, 5]

San Bernardino
San Bernardino County
Medical Center [5]

San Bernardino Valley
College [6]

San Bruno
Skyline College [6]

San Diego
Naval School of Health
Sciences [5]
San Diego Mesa College
[5]
University Hospital of San
Diego County [4]

San Francisco
City College of San
Francisco [4, 5]
College of California
Medical Affiliates [3, 7]
Pacific Medical Center—
Presbyterian Hospital
[2]
University of California—
San Francisco [5]

San Jose
O'Connor Hospital [5]

San Lorenzo
San Lorenzo Unified Sch.
Dist./Eden Area
Program [7]

Santa Ana
American College of
Paramedical Arts and
Sciences [3]

Santa Barbara
Cancer Foundation of
Santa Barbara [2]
Santa Barbara City College
[5]

Santa Monica
Santa Monica College [6]
Santa Monica Hospital
Medical Center [5]

Santa Rosa
Santa Rosa Junior College
[5, 6]

Sepulveda
Veterans Administration
Hospital [5]

Simi Valley
Simi Valley Adult School
[3]

South Laguna
South Coast Community
Hospital [5]

Stanford
Stanford University
Hospital & Clinic [4]

Stockton
San Joaquin General
Hospital [5]

Torrance
El Camino College [5, 6]
Los Angeles County—
Harbor General
Hospital [4]

Van Nuys
Los Angeles Valley
College [6]

Visalia
Kaweah Delta District
Hospital [5]

Walnut
Mt. San Antonio College
[5, 6]

Whittier
Rio Hondo College [6]

COLORADO

Aurora
Aurora Technical Center
[7]

Colorado Springs
Memorial Hospital [5]
Penrose Hospital [2]
St. Francis Hospital [5]

Denver
Community College of
Denver-Auraira
Campus [2, 4, 5, 6]
Presbyterian Medical
Center [5]
St. Anthony Hospital
Systems [2, 5]

Grand Junction
Mesa College [5]

Greeley
Weld County General
Hospital [5]

Pueblo
University of Southern
Colorado [5, 6]

CONNECTICUT

Bridgeport
Bridgeport Hospital [5, 7]
St. Vincent's Medical
Center [2, 5, 6]

Bristol
Bristol Hospital [5]

Danbury
Danbury Hospital [3, 5]

Hamden
Quinnipiac College [5]

Hartford
Hartford Hospital [5]
Mt. Sinai Hospital [5]
St. Francis Hospital [5, 7]

Manchester
Manchester Community
College [3, 6]
Manchester Memorial
Hospital [5]

Meriden
The Meriden-Wallingford
Hospital [5]

Middletown
Middlesex Community
College [5]

New Britain
New Britain General
Hospital [5]

New Haven
Hospital of St. Raphael
[5, 6]
South Central Community
College [4, 5]
Yale-New Haven Hospital
[2, 6]

New London
Lawrence and Memorial
Hospitals [5]

Norwalk
Norwalk Hospital [6]

Stamford
Stamford Hospital [5]

Waterbury
Mattatuck Community
College [5]
St. Mary's Hospital [7]

Willimantic
Windham Community
Memorial Hospital [5]

DELAWARE

Wilmington
Delaware Technical
Community College [6]
St. Francis Hospital, Inc.
[5]
Wilmington Medical
Center [5]

WASHINGTON, D.C.

George Washington
University Medical
Center [4]
Georgetown University
Hospital [5]
Howard University [4]
Howard University
Hospital [5]
Washington Hospital
Medical Center [5]
Washington Technical
Institute [5, 6]

FLORIDA

Boca Raton
Boca Raton Community
Hospital, Inc. [7]

Bradenton
Manatee Junior College
[5]
Manatee Memorial
Hospital [5]

Clearwater
Morton F. Plant Hospital
[5]

Coca
Brevard Community
College [5]

Daytona Beach
Daytona Beach
Community College [3]
Halifax Hospital Medical
Center [5]

Ft. Lauderdale
Broward Community
College [5, 6]

Ft. Myers
Lee Memorial Hospital [5]

Ft. Pierce
Indian River Community
College [5]

Gainesville
Santa Fe Community
College [2, 5, 6]
Veterans Administration
Hospital [1]

Hollywood
Broward Community
College [4]

Jacksonville
Baptist Memorial Hospital
[5]
Florida Junior College [6]
St. Luke's Hospital [5]
St. Vincent's Medical
Center [5]
University Hospital of
Jacksonville [5]

Lakeland
Lakeland General Hospital
[5]

Miami
University of Miami/
Jackson Memorial
Medical Center [2, 5]

Miami Beach
Miami-Dade Community
College [5, 6]

Mt. Sinai Medical Center
[2, 5]

North Miami
North Miami General
Hospital [5]

Orlando
Florida Hospital [5]
Florida Technological
University [5, 6]
Orange Memorial Hospital
[5]
Valencia Community
College [6]

Pensacola
Baptist Hospital [3]
Pensacola Junior College
[7]
Sacred Heart Hospital [5]
West Florida Medical
Center Clinic [5]

Sanford
Seminole Memorial
Hospital [5]

St. Petersburg
Bayfront Medical Center,
Inc. [5]
Florida Anesthesia
Services [7]
St. Petersburg Junior
College [6]
St. Petersburg Vocational-
Technical Institute [7]

Tallahassee
Tallahassee Community
College [5]

Tampa
Brewster Adult Technical
School [3]
Hillsborough Community
College [2, 5]
St. Joseph's Hospital

West Palm Beach
St. Mary's Hospital [5]

Winter Park
Winter Park Memorial
Hospital [5]

GEORGIA

Albany
Phoebe Putney Memorial
Hospital [5]

Atlanta
Crawford W. Long
Memorial Hospital [5]
Emory University [2, 5,
6, 7]
Georgia Baptist Hospital
[5]
Georgia State University
[6]
Grady Memorial Hospital
[2, 4]
Piedmont Hospital, Inc.
[5]
Medical College of
Georgia [2, 4, 5]

Brunswick
Brunswick Junior College
[5]

Clarkston
De Kalb Community
College [3]

Columbus
Medical Center [5]

Dalton
Hamilton Memorial
Hospital [5]

Decatur
De Kalb General Hospital
[2, 5]

Griffin
Griffin-Spaulding County
Hospital [5]

LaGrange
West Georgia Medical
Center [5]

Macon
Medical Center of Central
Georgia [5]

Marietta
Kennestone Hospital [5]

Milledgeville
Baldwin County Hospital
[5]

Rome
Floyd Hospital [5]

Savannah
Candler General Hospital,
Inc. [5]
Memorial Medical Center
[3, 5, 7]

Thomasville
Thomas Area Vocational
Technical School [7]

Valdosta
Valdosta Area Vocational-
Technical School [5]

Waycross
Waycross Memorial
Hospital [5]

HAWAII

Honolulu
Kapiolani Community
College [5]

IDAHO

Boise
Boise State University
[3, 5, 6]
St. Luke's Hospital, Ltd.
& Mountain States
Tumor Institute [4, 7]

Caldwell
Caldwell Memorial
Hospital [7]

Pocatello
Idaho State University [5]

ILLINOIS

Arlington Heights
Northwest Community
Hospital [5]

Belleville
Belleville Area College
[3, 5]

Centralia
St. Mary's Hospital [5]

Champaign
Parkland College [3, 5,
6, 7]

Chicago
Central YMCA
Community College
[5, 6]
Cook County Hospital [5]
De Paul University [5]
Henrotin Hospital [5]
Illinois Masonic Medical
Center [5]
Louis A. Weiss Memorial
Hospital [5]
Malcolm X College [5, 6]
Michael Reese Hospital &
Medical Center [5]
Northwestern Memorial
Hospital [2, 7]
Northwestern University
Medical Center [6]
Provident Hospital &
Training School [5]
Ravenswood Hospital
Medical Center [5]
Rush Presbyterian-St.
Luke's Medical Center
[4]
South Chicago Community
Hospital [5]
St. Anne's Hospital [5]
St. Joseph's Hospital [5]
St. Mary of Nazareth
Hospital Center [2, 5]
University of Chicago
Hospitals & Clinics
[6, 7]
University of Illinois
Hospital [5]
Woodlawn Hospital [5]
Wright Junior College [5]

Danville
LakeView Medical Center
[5]

Decatur
Decatur-Macon County
Hospital [5]

Dixon
Sauk Valley College [5]

East Peoria
Illinois Central College
[3, 5]

Elgin
St. Joseph Hospital [4, 5]

Evanston
Evanston Hospital [2, 4]
St. Francis Hospital [5]

Galesburg
Carl Sandburg College [5]

Glen Ellyn
College of Du Page [5]

Grayslake
College of Lake County
[5]

Hines
Edward Hines, Jr. Veterans
Administration Hospital
[2, 4]

Hinsdale
Hinsdale Sanitarium &
Hospital [5]

Kankakee
Kankakee Community
College [5]

Kewanee
Kewanee Public Hospital
[5]

Macomb
McDonough District
Hospital [5]

Malta
Kishwaukee College [5]

Moline
Lutheran Hospital [4, 5,
6, 7]
Moline Public Hospital
[3, 5]

Morton Grove
Oakton Community
College [5]

Normal
Bloomington-Normal
School of Radiologic
Technology [5]

Olney
Richland Memorial
Hospital [5]

Palos Hills
Moraine Valley
Community College
[3, 5, 6, 7]

Park Ridge
Lutheran General Hospital
[2]

Peoria
St. Francis Hospital [5]

Quincy
Blessing Hospital [3, 5]
St. Mary Hospital [5, 7]

River Grove
Triton College [2, 3, 5, 6]

Rock Island
Rock Island Franciscan
Hospital [5]

Rockford
Rockford Memorial
Hospital [5]
St. Anthony Hospital [6]
Swedish-American
Hospital [4, 5, 7]

South Holland
Thornton Community
College [5]

Springfield
Lincoln Land Community
College [5]
Memorial Medical Center
[5, 6]
St. John's Hospital [7]

Waukegan
Victory Memorial
Hospital [7]

INDIANA

Dyer
Our Lady of Mercy
Hospital [2]

East Chicago
St. Catherine Hospital [5]

Elkhart
Elkhart General Hospital
[5]

Evansville
Deaconess Hospital, Inc.
[6]
Evansville School of
Health Occupations [3]
Indiana State University at
Evansville [5]
University of Evansville
[5]
Welborn Memorial Baptist
Hospital [5]

Fort Wayne
Lutheran Hospital [5]
Parkview Memorial
Hospital [5]
St. Joseph's Hospital of
Fort Wayne, Inc. [5]

Gary
Indiana University,
Northwest Campus [6]
Indiana Vocational
Technical College-
Northwest Technical
Institute [3, 7]

Greenfield
Hancock County
Memorial Hospital [5]

Indianapolis
Community Hospital of
Indianapolis [2]
Indiana University School
of Medicine [2, 4, 5, 6]
Indiana Vocational
Technical College [3,
5, 7]
Methodist Hospital of
Indiana, Inc. [2, 7]

Kokomo
St. Joseph Memorial
Hospital [5]

Lafayette
Indiana Vocational
Technical College [3, 7]

Michigan City
Northern Indiana School
of Radiologic
Technology, Inc. [5]

Muncie
Ball Memorial Hospital
Association, Inc. [5]

Richmond
Reid Memorial Hospital
[5]

South Bend
Indiana Vocational
Technical College [3]
Memorial Hospital of
South Bend [5]

Valparaiso
Porter Memorial Hospital
[5]

Vincennes
Good Samaritan Hospital
[5]
Vincennes University [6]

IOWA

Ankeny
Des Moines Area
Community College [6]

Bettendorf
Scott Community College
[5]

Cedar Rapids
Kirkwood Community
College [6]
St. Luke's Methodist
Hospital [5]

Council Bluffs
Jennie Edmundson
Memorial Hospital [5]

Davenport
Scott Community College
[3]

Des Moines
Iowa Lutheran Hospital
[5]
Iowa Methodist Medical
Center [5]
Mercy Hospital [5]

Dubuque
Finley Hospital [5]
Mercy Medical Center [5]
Northeast Area One
Vocational Technical
School [7]

Iowa City
Mercy Hospital [5]
University of Iowa College
of Medicine [2]
University of Iowa
Hospitals & Clinics
[4, 5]

Mason City
St. Joseph Mercy
Hospital [5]

Ottumwa
Ottumwa Heights College
[5]

Sioux City
St. Joseph Mercy Hospital
[5]
St. Vincent Hospital [5]

Waterloo
Allen Memorial Hospital
[5]
Schoitz Memorial Hospital
[5]
St. Francis Hospital [5]

KANSAS

Garden City
St. Catherine Hospital
[2, 5]

Hays
Fort Hays State University
[5]

Hesston
Hesston College [6]

Hutchinson
Hutchinson Community
Junior College [5]

Kansas City
Bethany Medical Center
[5, 7]
Providence-St. Margaret
Health Center [5]
University of Kansas
Medical Center [2, 4,
5, 6]

Parsons
Labette Community
Junior College [5]

Topeka
St. Francis Hospital [5]
Stormont-Vail Hospital
[3, 5]

Wichita
St. Francis Hospital [2, 5]
St. Joseph Medical Center
[5]
Wesley Medical Center
[2, 3, 5]
Wichita State University
[6]

KENTUCKY

Ashland
King's Daughter's Hospital
[5]

Barbourville
Union College [5]

Covington
William Booth Memorial
Hospital [5]

Henderson
Community Methodist
Hospital [5]

Lexington
Central Baptist Hospital
[3, 5]
Good Samaritan Hospital
[5]

Lexington Technical
Institute/Univ. of
Kentucky [6]
St. Joseph Hospital [5, 7]
University of Kentucky
Medical Center [4, 5]

Louisville
Kentucky Baptist Hospital
[5]
Louisville General
Hospital [2, 5, 7]
Saints Mary & Elizabeth
Hospital [5]
U of KY/Jefferson
Community College/U
of Louisville Health
Sciences Ctr. [6]

Madisonville
Madisonville Area
Vocational School [5]

Morehead
Morehead State University
[5]

Owensboro
Owensboro-Daviess
County Hospital School
of Radiologic
Technology [5]

Paducah
Lourdes Hospital [5]

LOUISIANA

Alexandria
St. Frances Cabrini
Hospital [5]

Bastrop
Morehouse General
Hospital [5]

Baton Rouge
Earl K. Long Memorial
Hospital [7]

Bossier City
Bossier City General
Hospital [7]

Houma
Terrebonne General
Hospital [7]

Independence
Lallie Kemp Charity
Hospital/La. Health &
Human Resources
Administration [5]

Lafayette
Lafayette Charity Hospital
[5]
Our Lady of Lourdes
Hospital [5]

Monroe
St. Francis Hospital [5]

New Orleans
Alton Ochsner Medical
Foundation [2, 5, 6, 7]
Charity Hospital of
Louisiana at New
Orleans [2, 3, 5]
Delgado College [5, 6, 7]
Hotel Dieu Hospital [5]
Louisiana State University
Medical Center [1]
Methodist Hospital [5]
Sara Mayo Hospital [7]
St. Mary's Dominican
College [6]

Shreveport
Confederate Memorial
Medical Center [5]
Schumpert Medical Center
[5]
Veterans Administration
Hospital [2]

MAINE

Augusta
Augusta General Hospital
[5]

Bangor
Eastern Maine Vocational
Technical Institute [5]

Lewiston
Central Maine General
Hospital [5]

St. Mary's General
Hospital [5]

Portland
Maine Medical Center [5]
Mercy Hospital [5]

Waterville
Mid-Maine Medical
Center-Seton Unit [5]

MARYLAND

Baltimore
Baltimore City Hospitals
[5]
Community College of
Baltimore [6]
Essex Community College
[5]
Greater Baltimore Medical
Center [5]
Johns Hopkins Medical
Institutions [2, 4, 5]
Maryland General
Hospital [5]
Mercy Hospital, Inc. [5]
Provident Hospital
Complex [5]
Sinai Hospital of
Baltimore [5, 7]
South Baltimore General
Hospital [5]
University of Maryland
[5]

Bethesda
Naval Health Sciences
Education & Training
Command [2]

Cheverly
Prince George's General
Hospital [2]

Easton
The Memorial Hospital at
Easton [5]

Hagerstown
Hagerstown Junior
College [5]

Largo
Prince George's
Community College [5]

Salisbury
Peninsula General
Hospital [5, 7]

Takoma Park
Columbia Union College
[6]
Montgomery College [5]
Washington Adventist
Hospital [5]

MASSACHUSETTS

Bedford
Middlesex Community
College [5]

Beverly
Beverly Hospital [5]
North Shore Community
College [5]

Boston
Faulkner Hospital [5]
Harvard Joint Center for
Radiation Therapy [4]
Massachusetts General
Hospital [5, 7]
Northeastern University
[6]
Northeastern University at
Lincoln College [5]

Cambridge
Mount Auburn Hospital
[5]

Charlestown
Bunker Hill Community
College [5]

Fitchburg
Burbank Hospital [5]

Haverhill
Northern Essex
Community College
[5, 6, 7]

Holliston
Holliston Junior College
[7]

Holyoke
Holyoke Community
College [5]

New Bedford
St. Luke's Hospital [7]

North Adams
North Adams Regional
Hospital [5]

Quincy
Quincy Vocational
Technical School [3]

Salem
Salem Hospital [5]

Springfield
Springfield Technical
Community College [2,
4, 5, 6]

Stoughton
Goddard Memorial
Hospital [5]

Watertown
Massachusetts Bay
Community College [5]

Worcester
Quinsigamond Community
College [5, 6]

MICHIGAN

Ann Arbor
University of Michigan
Medical Center [2, 4]
Washtenaw Community
College [4, 5, 6]

Battle Creek
Kellogg Community
College [5]

Bay City
Delta College [5]
Mercy Hospital [5]

Benton Harbor
Lake Michigan College [5]

Big Rapids
Ferris State College [2, 5,
6]

Dearborn
Oakwood Hospital [5]

Detroit
Detroit General Hospital
[2, 5]
Detroit-Macomb Hospitals
Assn. [2, 5, 6]
Henry Ford Hospital [2, 5]
Mt. Carmel Mercy
Hospital & Medical
Center [5, 7]
St. John's Hospital [5, 7]
St. Joseph Mercy Hospital
[5]
United Hospitals of
Detroit [5]
University of Detroit [6]
Wayne State University
[4]

Eloise
Wayne County General
Hospital [5]

Flint
Hurley Medical Center [5]
McLaren General Hospital
[5]
St. Joseph Hospital [5]

Grand Rapids
Grand Rapids Junior
College [5]
St. Mary's Hospital [5]

Highland Park
Highland Park Community
College [6]

Jackson
W. A. Foote Memorial
Hospital, Inc. [5]

Kalamazoo
Borgess Hospital [5]
Bronson Methodist
Hospital [5]
Kalamazoo Valley
Community College [7]

Lansing
Lansing Community
College [5, 6, 7]

Livonia
St. Mary Hospital [5]

Mt. Clements
St. Joseph Hospital [5]

Muskegon
Hackley Hospital [5]

Petoskey
North Central Michigan
College [6]

Pontiac
St. Joseph Mercy Hospital
[5]

Port Huron
Port Huron Hospital [5]

Royal Oak
William Beaumont
Hospital [2, 4, 5]

Southfield
Providence Hospital [5]

Wayne
Annapolis Hospital [5]

MINNESOTA

Albert Lea
Naeve Hospital
Association [5]

Austin
St. Olaf Hospital [5]

Coon Rapids
Anoka-Hennepin Area
Vocational Technical
Institute [3, 7]

Crookston
Riverview Hospital
Association [5]

Detroit Lakes
St. Mary's Hospital [5]

Duluth
St. Luke's Hospital [5]
St. Mary's Hospital [5]

Hibbing
Hibbing General Hospital
[5]

Litchfield
Meeker County Memorial
Hospital [5]

Minneapolis
Abbott-Northwestern
  Hospital, Inc. [5]
Fairview Hospital [5]
Hennepin County Medical
  Center [2, 5]
Lutheran Deaconess
  Hospital [5]
Metropolitan Medical
  Center [5]
North Hennepin
  Community College [6]
North Memorial Medical
  Center [5]
St. Mary's Junior College
  [6]
University of Minnesota
  Health Sciences Center
  [4, 5]
University of Minnesota
  Hospitals [6]
Veterans Administration
  Hospital [2, 5]

Rochester
Mayo Foundation [2]
Rochester Area Vocational
  Technical Institute [3]
Rochester State
  Community College–
  Mayo Clinic [6]

St. Cloud
St. Cloud Hospital [5]

St. Louis Park
Methodist Hospital [5]

St. Paul
Bethesda Lutheran
  Hospital [5]
St. Joseph's Hospital [5]

Virginia
Virginia Municipal
  Hospital [5]

Willmar
Rice Memorial Hospital
  [5]

MISSISSIPPI

Gautier
Mississippi Gulf Coast Jr.
  College [5]

Greenville
King's Daughter Hospital
  [5]

Hattiesburg
Forrest County General
  Hospital-Methodist
  Hospital [5]
Pearl River Jr. College/
  Hattiesburg Voc/Tech
  [7]

Jackson
Mississippi Medical Center
  [5]
University of Mississippi
  Medical Center [2, 5]

Laurel
Jones County Community
  Hospital [5]

Meridan
Meridan Junior College
  [5, 7]

Raymond
Hinds Junior College [6, 7]

MISSOURI

Bridgeton
DePaul Community
  Health Center-DePaul
  Hospital [5]

Cape Girardeau
St. Francis Medical
  Center [2, 5]

Clayton
St. Louis County Hospital
  [5]

Columbia
Ellis Fischel State Cancer
  Hospital [4]
Harry S. Truman
  Memorial Veterans
  Hospital [2]
University of Missouri
  Medical Center-
  Columbia School of
  Medicine [4, 5, 6]

Independence
Independence Sanitorium
  & Hospital [5]

Joplin
Missouri Southern State
  College [5]

Kansas City
Baptist Memorial Hospital
  [5, 6]
Kansas City Technical
  Institute [3]
Menorah Medical Center
  [2, 5]
North Kansas City
  Memorial Hospital [5]
Penn Valley Community
  College [5]
Research Hospital &
  Medical Center [2, 5]
St. Luke's Hospital of
  Kansas City [2, 4, 5]

Lebanon
Louise G. Wallace
  Hospital [5]

Sedalia
State Fair Community
  College [7]

Springfield
Lester E. Cox Medical
  Center [5]
St. John's Hospital [5, 6]

St. Joseph
Methodist Medical Center
  [5]

St. Louis
Homer G. Phillips Hospital
  [5]
Mallinckrodt Institute of
  Radiology-Washington
  University [2, 4]
Maryville College of the
  Sacred Heart [6]
St. John's Mercy Medical
  Center [2, 5]
St. Louis Community
  College at Forest Park
  [5, 6]

Veterans Administration
Hospital [2]
Washington University
School of Medicine [5]

MONTANA

Billings
St. Vincent's Hospital [5]

Great Falls
Columbus Hospital [5]
Montana Deaconess Medi-
cal Center [5]

Missoula
St. Patrick Hospital [5]

NEBRASKA

Grand Island
St. Francis Hospital [5]

Hastings
Mary Lanning Memorial
Hospital [5]

Lincoln
Bryan Memorial Hospital
[7]
Southeast Community
College [3, 5]

Omaha
Archbishop Bergan Mercy
Hospital [5]
College of Saint Mary [6]
Creighton Memorial-
St. Joseph Hospital [5]
Immanuel Medical Center
[5, 6]
University of Nebraska
College of Medicine
[2, 4, 5]

Scottsbluff
West Nebraska General
Hospital [5]

NEVADA

Henderson
Rose de Lima Hospital [5]

Las Vegas
University of Nevada [5]

Reno
Washoe Medical Center
[4]
Western Nevada
Community College [5]

NEW HAMPSHIRE

Concord
New Hampshire Technical
Institute [5]

Keene
Cheshire Hospital [5]

Laconia
Lakes Region General
Hospital [5]

Manchester
Elliot Hospital [5]

Nashua
Nashua Hospital
Association (Memorial
Hospital) [5]

NEW JERSEY

Atlantic City
Atlantic City Medical
Center [2, 5]

Bayonne
Bayonne Hospital [5]

Belleville
Clara Maass Memorial
Hospital [5]

Bridgeton
Bridgeton Hospital [5]

Camden
Cooper Hospital [2, 5]
Our Lady of Lourdes
Hospital [5]
West Jersey Hospital,
Northern Division [5]

Cape May Court House
Burdette Tomlin Memorial
Hospital [5]

Cherry Hill
Institute for Advancement
of Medical Sciences
[3, 5]

East Orange
Veterans Administration
Hospital [2]

Edison
John F. Kennedy Medical
Center [2]
Middlesex County College
[5]

Elizabeth
Elizabeth General Hospital
& Dispensary [5]

Englewood
Englewood Hospital
Association [5]

Flemington
Hunterdon Medical
Center [5]

Hackensack
Hackensack Hospital [5]

Jersey City
Christ Hospital [5]
Jersey City Medical
Center [5, 7]

Lincroft
Brookdale Community
College [6]

Livingston
St. Barnabas Medical
Center [2, 4, 5]

Long Branch
Monmouth Medical
Center [2, 4, 5]

Madison
Fairleigh Dickinson
University [5, 6]

Mays Landing
Atlantic Community
College [6]

Montclair
Mountainside Hospital [5]

Mt. Holly
Burlington County
Memorial Hospital
[5, 7]

Newark
Essex County College [5]
Harrison S. Martland
Hospital [5]
New Jersey Medical
School/College of
Medicine & Dentistry of
NJ [7]
St. Michael's Medical
Center [5]

Orange
Hospital Center of Orange
[2]

Paramus
Bergen Community
College [5, 6]

Passaic
Passaic General Hospital
[5]
Passaic County
Community College
[5, 7]
St. Joseph's Hospital and
Medical Center [2]

Plainfield
Muhlenberg Hospital [5]

Red Bank
Riverview Hospital [5]

Ridgewood
Valley Hospital [5]

Scotch Plains
Union County Technical
Institute [6]

Summit
Overlook Hospital [2, 4, 5]

Trenton
Helene Fuld Hospital [5]
Mercer County
Community College [5]
Mercer Medical Center [2]
St. Francis Medical
Center [5]

Turnersville
Washington Memorial
Hospital [2]

Westwood
Pascack Valley Hospital
[5]

NEW MEXICO

Albuquerque
Albuquerque Technical-
Vocational Institute [7]
University of Albuquerque
[5, 6]
University of New Mexico
School of Medicine [2, 5]

Carlsbad
Carlsbad Regional
Medical Center [5]

Hobbs
Llano Estacado Medical
Center [5]

Las Cruces
Dona-Ana County
Occupational Education
[5]

NEW YORK

Albany
Albany Medical Center
Hospital [5]
Memorial Hospital [5]

Binghamton
Broome Community
College [5]

Bronx
Hostos Community
College [5]
Misericordia Hospital
Medical Center [5]
Montefiore Hospital &
Medical Center [4, 5]

Brooklyn
Long Island College
Hospital [5]

Long Island University/
The Brooklyn Center [6]
New York City
Community College [5]
The Brooklyn Hospital [2]

Buffalo
Erie Community College
[4, 6]
Millard Fillmore Hospital
[5]
Trocaire College [5]

Cambridge
Mary McClellan Hospital
[5]

Corning
Corning Hospital [5]

East Meadow
Nassau County Medical
Center [2, 6]

Elmira
Arnot-Ogden Memorial
Hospital [5]
Elmira College [7]
St. Joseph's Hospital
Health Center [5]

Far Rockaway
Peninsula Hospital Center
[2, 5]

Garden City
Nassau Community
College [3, 5]

Glen Cove
Community Hospital at
Glen Cove [5]

Glens Falls
Glens Falls Hospital [5]

Greenvale
C. W. Post Center of
Long Island University
[5]

Hornell
St. James Mercy Hospital
[5]

Ithaca
Tompkins County
Hospital [5]

Jamaica
Catholic Medical Center
[5]

Jamestown
Woman's Christian
Association Hospital [5]

Johnson City
Charles S. Wilson
Memorial Hospital [7]

Lewiston
Mt. St. Mary's Hospital of
Niagara Falls [5]

Mineola
Nassau Hospital [5]

New York
Bellevue Hospital Center
[5]
Borough of Manhattan
Community College [6]
City of New York Hospital
Affiliate [7]
Columbia Presbyterian
Medical Center [1, 3, 5]
Flower-Fifth Ave.
Hospitals [5]
Harlem Hospital Center
[2]
Hospital for Joint
Diseases & Medical
Center [5]
Lenox Hill Hospital [6]
Memorial Hospital for
Cancer and Allied
Diseases [4, 5]
New York Hospital-
Cornell Medical Center
[5]
New York University
Medical Center [2, 6, 7]
St. Claire's Hospital &
Health Center [5]

Niagara Falls
Niagara Falls Memorial
Medical Center [5]

Northport
Veterans Administration
Hospital [2, 5]

Oceanside
South Nassau
Communities Hospital
[5]

Plattsburgh
Champlain Valley
Physicians Hospital
Medical Center [5]

Port Chester
United Hospital [1, 5]

Riverdale
Manhattan College [2]

Riverhead
Central Suffolk Hospital
[5]

Rochester
Genesee Hospital [5]
Monroe Community
College [5]
Rochester Institute of
Technology [2]

Rockville Centre
Mercy Hospital [5]

Saranac
North Country
Community College [5]

Staten Island
U.S. Public Health
Service [5]

Stony Brook
State University of N.Y.
at Stony Brook [6]

Syracuse
Onondaga Community
College [7]
State University of N.Y.-
Upstate Medical Center
[2, 4, 5, 6]

Troy
Hudson Valley
Community College
[5, 6]

Utica
St. Elizabeth Hospital [5]
St. Luke's Memorial
Hospital Center [5]

Valhalla
Westchester Community
College [5, 6]

NORTH CAROLINA

Albemarle
Stanly Technical Institute
[7]

Asheville
Asheville-Buncombe
Technical Institute [5]

Carthage
Sandhills Community
College [5]

Chapel Hill
North Carolina Memorial
Hospital [4]
University of North
Carolina [2, 5]

Charlotte
Central Piedmont
Community College [6]
Charlotte Memorial
Hospital and Medical
Center [5]
Mercy Hospital, Inc. [5]
Presbyterian Hospital [5]

Durham
Duke University Medical
Center [2, 5]
Durham County General
Hospital [5]
Durham Technical
Institute [6]

Elkin
Hugh Chatham Memorial
Hospital [5]

Fayetteville
Fayetteville Technical
Institute [3, 5]

Gastonia
Gaston Memorial
Hospital, Inc. [5]

Greensboro
Moses H. Cone Memorial
Hospital [5]

Greenville
Pitt Technical Institute [5]

Henderson
Maria Parham Hospital
Association, Inc. [5]

Hickory
Catawba Memorial
Hospital [5]

Kingston
Lenoir Memorial Hospital,
Inc. [5]

Lenoir
Caldwell Community
College [5]

Morehead City
Carteret Technical
Institute [5]

Mount Airy
Northern Hospital of
Surry County [5]

North Wilkesboro
Wilks General Hospital
[5]

Raleigh
Rex Hospital [5]

Salisbury
Rowan Technical Institute
[5]

Shelby
Cleveland County
Technical Institute [5]

Smithfield
Johnston Technical
Institute [5]

Statesville
Davis Hospital [5]
Iredell Memorial Hospital
[5]

Sylva
C. J. Harris Community
Hospital [5]

Tarboro
Edgecombe Technical
Institute [5]

Washington
Beaufort County Hospital
[5]

Winston-Salem
Forsyth Technical
Institute [2, 5, 6]

NORTH DAKOTA

Bismarck
Quain & Ramstad Clinic
[5]
St. Alexius Hospital [5, 6]

Fargo
St. John's Hospital [5]
St. Luke's Hospital [5, 7]

Grand Forks
United Hospital-Grand
Forks Clinic [5]

Minot
St. Joseph's Hospital [5]
Trinity Medical Center
[2, 5]

OHIO

Akron
Akron City Hospital [5]
Akron General Medical
Center [5]
Children's Hospital of
Akron [5]
St. Thomas Hospital [5]

Barberton
Barberton Citizens
Hospital [5]

Berea
Southwest General
Hospital [5]

Canton
Aultman Hospital
Association [2, 5, 7]
Timken Mercy Hospital
[5]

Cincinnati
Christ Hospital [4, 5]

Cincinnati Technical
College [7]
College of Mount St.
Joseph on the Ohio [7]
Our Lady of Mercy
Hospital [5]
University of Cincinnati
Medical Center [2, 5]
Xavier University [5]

Cleveland
Cleveland Clinic
Educational Foundation
[4]
Cleveland Metropolitan
General Hospital [5]
Hilcrest Hospital [2, 5]
Mt. Sinai Hospital of
Cleveland [5]
St. Alexis Hospital [5]
St. Luke's Hospital [5]
St. Vincent Charity
Hospital [2]
University Hospitals of
Cleveland [5]

Columbus
Columbus Public Schools
[7]
Columbus Technical
Institute [6]
Mt. Carmel Medical
Center [5, 7]
Ohio State University
College of Medicine
[5, 6]
Ohio State University
Hospital [2]
Riverside Methodist
Hospital [2, 5]

Cuyahoga Falls
Green Cross General
Hospital [5]

Dayton
Grandview Hospital [2]
Miami Valley Hospital
[2, 7]
Sinclair Community
College [5, 6]

Dover
Union Hospital [5]

Elyria
Lorain County
Community College [5]

Euclid
Euclid General Hospital
[5]

Garfield Heights
Marymount Hospital [5]

Hamilton
Fort Hamilton-Hughes
Memorial Hospital
Center [5]
Mercy Hospital [5]

Kettering
Kettering College of
Medical Arts [5, 6]
Kettering Medical Center
[7]

Lancaster
Lancaster-Fairfield
County Hospital [5]

Mansfield
North Central Technical
College [5]

Marietta
Memorial Hospital [5]

Marion
Marion General Hospital
[5]

Massillon
NEORAD Northeast Ohio
Radiation Oncology
Center [4]

Maumee
St. Luke's Hospital [5]

Middletown
Middletown Hospital
Association [5]

Newark
Central Ohio Technical
College [5]

Norwalk
Fisher-Titus Memorial
Hospital [5]

Parma
Cuyahoga Community
College [6]
Parma Community
General Hospital [5]

Perrysburg
Michael J. Ownes
Technical College [5]

Portsmouth
Shawnee State College [5]

Ravena
Robinson Memorial
Hospital [5]

Salem
Northern Columbiana
County Community
Hospital [5]

Sandusky
Providence Hospital [5]

Springfield
Community Hospital of
Springfield & Clark
County [5]
Wittenberg University [5]

Steubenville
Ohio Valley Hospital [5]

Tiffin
Mercy Hospital [5]

Toledo
St. Vincent Hospital &
Medical Center [5]
The Toledo Hospital [5]
University of Toledo
Community &
Technical College [6, 7]

Warren
Trumbull Memorial
Hospital [5]

Youngstown
St. Elizabeth Hospital [2,
5, 7]
Youngstown Hospital
Association-North Unit
[5]

Youngstown Hospital
Association-South Unit
[5]

Zanesville
Bethesda Hospital
Association [5]
Muskingum Area Joint
Vocational School for
Adult Education [7]

OKLAHOMA

Enid
St. Mary's Hospital [5]

Midwest City
Oscar Rose Junior College
[5, 6]

Oklahoma City
Baptist Medical Center of
Oklahoma [5, 7]
Mercy Health Center [5]
Presbyterian Hospital [5]
University of Oklahoma
Health Sciences Center
[2, 4, 5]

Tulsa
Hillcrest Medical Center
[2, 5]
St. Francis Hospital [2, 4]
Tulsa Junior College [5, 6]

OREGON

Albany
Albany General Hospital
[5]

Eugene
Lane Community College
[6]

Grants Pass
Rogue Community
College [7]

Gresham
Mt. Hood Community
College [6]

Klamath Falls
Oregon Institute of
Technology [5]

Portland
Portland Community
College [5]
University of Oregon
Health Sciences Center
[4]

PENNSYLVANIA

Abington
Abington Memorial
Hospital [5]

Aliquippa
Aliquippa Hospital [5]

Allentown
Allentown Hospital
Association [5]

Altoona
Altoona Hospital [5]
Mercy Hospital [5]

Beaver Falls
Medical Center of Beaver
County, Inc. [5]

Bethlehem
Northampton County
Area Community
College [5]

Bryn Mawr
Bryn Mawr Hospital [5, 7]

Camp Hill
Holy Spirit Hospital [5]

Carlisle
Carlisle Hospital [5]

Chester
Crozier-Chester Medical
Center [5, 6]
Sacred Heart General
Hospital [5]

Coatesville
Coatesville Hospital [5]

Dallas
College Misericordia [5]

Danville
Geisinger Medical Center
[4, 5]

Darby
Mercy Catholic Medical
Center [5]

Doylestown
Doylestown Hospital [5]

Elkins Park
Rolling Hill Hospital &
Diagnostic Center [5]

Eire
Hamot Medical Center
[5, 7]
St. Vincent Health Center
[5]

Franklin
Franklin Hospital [5]

Gwynedd Valley
Gwynedd Mercy Hospital
[4]

Harrisburg
Harrisburg Hospital [2, 5]
Harrisburg Polyclinic
Hospital [2, 5]

Hazleton
St. Joseph Hospital [5]

Hershey
Milton S. Hershey Medical
Center Hospital [4, 5]

Jeannette
Monsour Hospital and
Clinic [5]

Johnstown
Conemaugh Valley
Memorial Hospital
[3, 5]
Lee Hospital [5]

Kittanning
Armstrong County
Memorial Hospital [5]

Lancaster
Lancaster General
Hospital [2, 5]
St. Joseph Hospital [5, 6]

McKees Rocks
Ohio Valley General
Hospital [5]

McKeesport
McKeesport Hospital [5]

Meadowbrook
Holy Redeemer Hospital
[5]

Natrona Heights
Allegheny Valley Hospital
[5]

Norristown
Montgomery Hospital [5]
Sacred Heights Hospital
[5]

Philadelphia
Albert Einstein Medical
Center-Northern
Division [5]
Chestnut Hill Hospital [5]
Community College of
Philadelphia [5, 6]
Episcopal Hospital [5]
Germantown Dispensary
& Hospital [5]
Graduate Hospital of the
University of
Pennsylvania [5]
Hahnemann Medical
College & Hospital
[5, 6]
Hospital of the University
of Pennsylvanaia [5, 7]
James Martin School/
Adult Educational
Training Center [7]
Lankenau Hospital [5]
Medical College of
Pennsylvania [5]
Mercy Catholic Medical
Center [7]
Murrell Dobbins Area
Vocational Technical
School [5]
Nazareth Hospital [5]
St. Joseph's Hospital [5]
Temple University [5]
Temple University
Medical Center [2]
Thomas Jefferson
University [5]
Veterans Administration
Hospital [5]

Pittsburgh
Allegheny General
Hospital [4]
Community College of
Allegheny County [6]
Indiana University of
Pennsylvania/Western
Pennsylvania Hospital
[6]
Mercy Hospital of
Pittsburgh [5]
Montefiore Hospital [5]
Presbyterian-University
Hospital [4, 5]
Robert Morris College [5]
Shadyside Hospital [5]
St. Francis General
Hospital [7]
Western Pennsylvania
Hospital [5]

Pottsville
Pottsville Hospital &
Warne Clinic [5]

Reading
Community General
Hospital [5]
Reading Hospital and
Medical Center [5]
St. Joseph's Hospital [5]

Sayre
Robert Packer Hospital
[3, 6]

Scranton
Community Medical
Center [5]
Scranton State General
Hospital [5]

Sewickley
Sewickley Valley Hospital
[5]

Sharon
Sharon General Hospital
[5]

Somerset
Somerset Community
Hospital [5]

Washington
Washington Hospital [5]

Waynesburg
Greene County Memorial
Hospital [5]

Wilkes-Barre
Wilkes-Barre General
Hospital [5]

Williamsport
Williamsport Area
Community College [5]

York
York Hospital [2, 5, 7]

RHODE ISLAND

Lincoln
Rhode Island Junior
College [5]

Providence
Rhode Island Hospital
[2, 6, 7]

SOUTH CAROLINA

Anderson
Anderson Memorial
Hospital [5]
McDuffie Vocational High
School [3]

Charleston
Medical University of
South Carolina [5, 6]

Columbia
Midlands Technical
College [5, 6]
Richland Memorial
Hospital [2]
South Carolina Baptist
Hospital [5]

Florence
McLeod Memorial
Hospital [5]

Greenville
Greenville Technical
College [3, 5, 6]

Greenwood
Greenwood County
Vocational Facilities [7]

Piedmont Technical
College [5]
Self Memorial Hospital [2]

Orangeburg
Orangeburg-Calhoun TEC
College [5]

Rock Hill
York General Hospital [5]

Spartanburg
Spartanburg Technical
College [3, 5]

SOUTH DAKOTA

Aberdeen
St. Luke's Hospital [5]

Mitchell
Dakota Wesleyan
University-St. Joseph
Hospital [5]

Rapid City
Rapid City, Regional
Hospital, Inc. [5]

Sioux Falls
McKennan Hospital [5, 6]
Sioux Valley Hospital [5, 6]

Yankton
Mount Marty College [6]
Sacred Heart Hospital [5]

TENNESSEE

Chattanooga
Baroness Erlanger
Hospital [6]
Chattanooga State
Technical Community
College [5]

Columbia
Columbia State
Community College [5]

Crossville
State Area Vocational
Technical School [5]

Elizabethton
Elizabethton Paramedical
  Vocational Technical
  School [5, 7]

Gallatin
Volunteer State
  Community College [7]

Harriman
Roane State Community
  College [5]

Jackson
Jackson State Community
  College [5, 6]

Knoxville
East Tennessee Baptist
  Hospital [5]
University of Tennessee
  Memorial Hospital [5]

Madison
Madison Hospital [5]

Maryville
Blount Memorial Hospital
  [5]

Memphis
Baptist Memorial Hospital
  [2, 4, 5, 6]
City of Memphis Hospitals
  [2]
Memphis Area Vocational-
  Technical School [7]
Methodist Hospital [4, 5,
  6]
St. Joseph Hospital [5]
University of Tennessee
  Center for the Health
  Sciences [5]

Nashville
Aquinas Junior College [5]
Nashville Metropolitan
  General Hospital [5]
Vanderbilt University
  Medical Center [4]
Vanderbilt University/
  Aquinas Junior College
  [6]

TEXAS

Abilene
Hendrick Memorial
  Hospital [5]

Amarillo
Amarillo College [5, 6]

Austin
Austin Community
  College [5]
Austin State Hospital [5]

Baytown
San Jacinto Methodist
  Hospital [5]

Beaumont
Lamar University [5, 7]
The Baptist Hospital of
  Southeast Texas, Inc. [5]

Big Spring
Malone and Hogan
  Hospital [5]

Brownsville
Texas Southmost College
  [5]

Corpus Christi
Del Mar College [3, 5, 6, 7]

Corsicana
Navarro County Memorial
  Hospital [5]

Dallas
Dallas County Hospital
  District [3]
El Centro College [5, 6, 7]
St. Paul Hospital [4]

El Paso
El Paso Community
  College [5, 6]

Fort Sam Houston
Brooke Army Medical
  Center [5, 7]

Fort Worth
Harris Hospital [7]
Radiation & Medical
  Research Foundation of
  the Southwest [4]

Galveston
University of Texas
  School of Allied Health
  Sciences/Galveston
  College [1, 5, 6]
University of Texas
  Medical Branch at
  Galveston [5]

Houston
Baylor College of
  Medicine [2, 4]
Ben Taub Hospital [3]
Houston Community
  College [3, 5, 6]
Memorial Hospital System
  [5]
Texas Southern University
  [6]

Hurst
Tarrant County Junior
  College [3, 5, 6]

Kermit
Memorial Hospital [5]

Laredo
Laredo Junior College [5]

Levelland
South Plains College [5]

Longview
The Good Shepherd
  Hospital [5]

Lubbock
Methodist Hospital [5]

Lufkin
Angelina College [5]
Memorial Hospital [5]

Odessa
Odessa College [5]

Pasadena
San Jacinto College [3, 5]

Plainview
Central Plains General
  Hospital [5]

San Antonio
Baptist Memorial Hospital
  [5]
St. Philip's College [5, 7]

San Marcos
Southwest Texas State
 University [6]

Snyder
D. M. Cogdell Memorial
 Hospital [5]

Temple
Scott & White Memorial
 Hospital [2]

Texarkana
Wadley Hospital [5]

Tyler
Tyler Junior College [5, 6]

Victoria
Citizens Memorial
 Hospital [5]

Waco
McLellan Community
 College [5]

Wichita Falls
Midwestern University [5]
USAF H.S. Military/
 Shephard Air Force
 Base [3, 5]

UTAH

Ogden
Weber State College [5, 6]

Provo
Utah Valley Hospital [5]

Salt Lake City
L.D.S. Hospital [4]
St. Mark's Hospital [5]
University of Utah [2]
University of Utah
 Medical Center [4, 5]

VERMONT

Burlington
University of Vermont
 [2, 4, 5]

Rutland
Rutland Hospital, Inc. [5]

VIRGINIA

Annandale
Northern Virginia
 Community College [6]

Big Stone Gap
Mountain Empire
 Community College [7]

Charlottesville
Piedmont Virginia
 Community College [6]
University of Virginia
 Medical Center [2, 4, 5]

Clifton Forge
Emmett Memorial
 Hospital [5]

Danville
The Memorial Hospital
 [5]

Falls Church
The Fairfax Hospital [5, 7]

Hampton
Hampton General
 Hospital [5]

Harrisonburg
Rockingham Memorial
 Hospital [5]

Lynchburg
Central Virginia
 Community College
 [5, 7]

Newport News
Newport News Public
 School and Riverside
 Hospital [3]
Riverside Hospital [5]

Norfolk
DePaul Hospital [5]
Medical Center Hospitals
 [4, 5]

Petersburg
Petersburg General
 Hospital [5]

Portsmouth
Maryview Hospital [5]
Naval Regional Medical
 Center [3, 5]

Richlands
Southwest Virginia
 Community College
 [5, 7]

Richmond
Medical College of
 Virginia/Virginia
 Commonwealth
 University [4, 5]
Richmond Memorial
 Hospital [5]
St. Mary's Hospital [5]

Roanoke
Roanoke Memorial
 Hospital [2, 4, 5]
Virginia Western
 Community College [5]

Suffolk
Louise Obici Memorial
 Hospital [5]

Virginia Beach
Tidewater Community
 College [7]

Winchester
Shenandoah College [6]
Winchester Memorial
 Hospital [5, 7]

WASHINGTON

Bellevue
Bellevue Community
 College [5]

Kent
Highline Community
 College [6]

Seattle
Seattle Central
 Community College [7]
Swedish Hospital Medical
 Center [2, 4, 5]

Spokane
Holy Family Hospital [2, 5]
Spokane Community College [6]

Tacoma
Tacoma Community College [5]

Wenatchee
Wenatchee Valley College [5]

Yakima
Yakima Valley College [5]

WEST VIRGINIA

Bluefield
Bluefield Sanitarium [5]

Charleston
Morris Harvey College [5]
St. Francis Hospital [5]

Clarksburg
United Hospital Center [5]

Elkins
Memorial General Hospital [5]

Fairmont
Fairmont General Hospital [5]

Huntington
St. Mary's Hospital [5]

Morgantown
West Virginia University Hospital [4, 5]

Parkersburg
Camden Clark Memorial Hospital [5]
Parkersburg Community College [5]

South Williamson
Williamson Appalachian Regional Hospital [5]

Weston
Stonewall Jackson Memorial Hospital [5]

Wheeling
Ohio Valley Medical Center, Inc. [5]
Wheeling Hospital [5]

WISCONSIN

Beloit
Beloit Memorial Hospital [5]

Cudahy
Trinity Memorial Hospital [5]

Eau Claire
District One Technical Institute [5]
Luther Hospital [5]

Fond Du Lac
St. Agnes Hospital [5]

Green Bay
Bellin Memorial Hospital [5]

Kenosha
Kenosha Memorial Hospital [5]
St. Catherine's Hospital [5]

La Crosse
Western Wisconsin Technical Institute [1, 3, 5]

Madison
Madison General Hospital [5]
St. Marys Hospital Medical Center [2, 5]
University of Wisconsin-Madison [4, 5]

Marshfield
Marshfield Medical Foundation [4]
St. Joseph's Hospital [5]

Milwaukee
Alverno College [2]
Columbia Hospital [5]

Deaconess Hospital [5]
Family Hospital [5]
Lutheran Hospital of Milwaukee, Inc. [5]
Medical College of Wisconsin [4]
Milwaukee Area Technical College [6]
Milwaukee County Medical Complex [2, 6]
St. Joseph's Hospital [5]
St. Luke's Hospital [2, 5]
St. Mary's Hospital [5]
St. Michael Hospital [5]

Neenah
Theda Clark Memorial Hospital [5]

Oshkosh
Mercy Medical Center [5]

Pewaukee
Waukesha County Technical Institute [3]

Racine
St. Luke's Memorial Hospital [5]
St. Mary's Hospital [5]

Rhinelander
St. Mary's Hospital [5]

Waukesha
Waukesha Memorial Hospital [5]

Wausau
North Central Technical Institute [5]

Wood
Veterans Administration Center [5]

WYOMING

Cheyenne
Laramie County Community College [5]

Cody
West Park County Hospital [5]

Educational Programs: Diagnostic Medical Ultrasound

ALABAMA

University of Southern Alabama
Mobile

CALIFORNIA

Bay General Community Hospital
Chula Vista

French Hospital and Medical Clinic
San Luis Obispo

Loma Linda University
Loma Linda

Martin Luther King, Jr. General Hospital
Los Angeles

Omnimedical Services, Inc.
Paramount

Santa Barbara Cottage Hospital
Santa Barbara

University of California at
   San Francisco Hospital
San Francisco

University of California, Los Angeles
   Hospital
Los Angeles

V. A. Wadsworth Hospital Center
Los Angeles

V. A. Hospital of San Diego
San Diego

COLORADO

University of Colorado Medical Center
Denver

CONNECTICUT

Yale University School of Medicine
New Haven

FLORIDA

Florida Medical Center
Lauderdale Lakes

Mt. Sinai Hospital
Miami

West Florida Hospital
Pensacola

ILLINOIS

Northwest Community Hospital
Arlington Heights

INDIANA

Methodist Hospital of Gary, Inc.
Gary

KANSAS

University of Kansas Hospital
Kansas City

MARYLAND

Maryland Institute of Ultrasound
Baltimore

MAINE

Maine Medical Center
Portland

MASSACHUSETTS

Middlesex Community College
Bedford

MICHIGAN

Henry Ford Hospital
Detroit

Oakwood Hospital
Dearborn

Providence Hospital
Southfield

NEW YORK

New York Hospital/Cornell Medical
   Center
New York City

New York Radiological Institute
New York City

State University Downstate Medical
   Center
Brooklyn

Upstate Medical Center Hospital
Syracuse

OHIO

Aultman Hospital
Canton

Mt. Sinai Hospital of Cleveland
Cleveland

OKLAHOMA

University of Oklahoma
Oklahoma City

PENNSYLVANIA

Jefferson University Medical Center
Philadelphia

Hospital of the University of Pennsylvania
Philadelphia

Westmoreland Hospital
Greensburg

WASHINGTON

School of Science & Engineering
Seattle University
Seattle

Swedish Hospital and Medical Center
Seattle

WISCONSIN

St. Mary's Hospital
Milwaukee

Educational Programs

CARDIOLOGY TECHNOLOGY

Programs listed have conditional approval by the American Cardiology Technologists Association.

Grossmont College
El Cajon, CA

University of Toledo
Community and Technical College
Toledo, OH

Penn Valley Community College
Kansas City, MO

Temple Junior College
Temple, TX

CARDIOPULMONARY TECHNOLOGY

Programs accredited by National Society for Cardiopulmonary Technology

Grossmont College
El Cajon, CA

Stony Brook University
Stony Brook, NY

Cardiopulmonary Technicians School
San Diego, CA

Santa Fe Community College
Gainesville, FL

Mercy Catholic Medical Center
Darby, PA

Cardiopulmonary Technicians School
Naval School of Health Sciences
Bethesda, MD

Spokane Community College
Spokane, WA

Educational Programs: Cardiovascular Perfusion

Programs accredited by the American Board of Cardiovascular Perfusion

Stanford University School of Medicine
Stanford, CA

V. A. Hospital
Long Beach, CA

Mount Sinai Hospital
Chicago, IL

State University of New York
Upstate Medical Center
Syracuse, NY

Ohio State University School of
  Allied Medical Professions
Columbus, OH

University of Oregon Health Sciences
  Center
Portland, OR

Shadyside School of Perfusion
Pittsburgh, PA

Medical University of South Carolina
Charleston, SC

Perfusion Associates
Houston, TX

Texas Heart Institute
Houston, TX

Educational Programs: Biomedical Engineering

University of Alabama—Birmingham
Birmingham, AL

Boston University
Boston, MA

Brown University
Providence, RI

California State University
Long Beach, CA

University of California
Berkeley, CA

University of California
Davis, CA

Carnegie-Mellon University
Pittsburgh, PA

Case Western Reserve University
Cleveland, OH

Catholic University of America
Washington, DC

Clemson University
Clemson, SC

Cleveland State University
Cleveland, OH

Columbia University
New York, NY

University of Connecticut
Storrs, CT

Drexel University
Philadelphia, PA

Duke University
Durham, NC

Fairleigh Dickinson University
Teaneck, NJ

Illinois Institute of Technology
Chicago, IL

University of Illinois at Chicago Circle
Chicago, IL

Iowa State University
Ames, IA

University of Iowa
Iowa City, IA

Johns Hopkins Medical School
Baltimore, MD

Louisiana Tech University
Ruston, LA

University of Louisville
Louisville, KY

Marquette University and Medical College
Milwaukee, WI

Massachusetts Institute of Technology
Cambridge, MA

University of Miami
Coral Gables, FL

University of Michigan
Ann Arbor, MI

Milwaukee School of Engineering
Milwaukee, WI

University of Minnesota
Minneapolis, MN

University of Mississippi
University, MS

University of New Mexico
Albuquerque, NM

Polytechnic Institute of New York
Brooklyn, NY

University of North Carolina
Chapel Hill, NC

Northwestern University
Evanston, IL

University of the Pacific
Stockton, CA

University of Pennsylvania
Philadelphia, PA

University of Pennsylvania
University Park, PA

Rensselaer Polytechnic Institute
Troy, NY

Rutgers University
New Brunswick, NJ

University of Southern California
Los Angeles, CA

Southern Methodist University
Dallas, TX

Syracuse University
Syracuse, NY

Temple University
Philadelphia, PA

Texas A & M University
College Station, TX

Texas Tech University
Lubbock, TX

University of Texas
Austin, TX

University of Texas at Arlington
Arlington, TX

Tulane University
New Orleans, LA

Vanderbilt University
Nashville, TN

University of Virginia
Charlottesville, VA

Wichita State University
Wichita, KS

University of Wisconsin
Madison, WI

Worcester Polytechnic Institute
Worcester, MA

University of Wyoming
Laramie, WY

Educational Programs:
Biomedical Equipment Technology*

Amarillo College
Amarillo, TX

Brevard Community College
Cocoa, FL

Brown Institute
Minneapolis, MN

Catonsville Community College
Catonsville, MD

Chattanooga State Technical Institute
Chattanooga, TN

College of the Desert
Palm Desert, CA

Colorado Technical College
Manitou Springs, CO

Franklin Institute of Boston
Boston, MA

Golden West College
Huntington Beach, CA

Grossmont College
El Cajon, CA

Kettering College of Medical Arts
Kettering, OH

Lincoln College, Northwestern University
Boston, MA

Los Angeles City College
Los Angeles, CA

Los Angeles Valley College
Van Nuys, CA

Michael J. Owens Technical College
Perrysburg, OH

Milwaukee Area Technical College
Milwaukee, WI

Monroe Community College
Rochester, NY

Regional Technical Institute
University of Alabama
Birmingham, AL

Schoolcraft College
Livonia, MI

School of Health Care Services
U.S. Air Force
Sheppard AFB, TX

Springfield Tech Community College
Springfield, MA

State Technical Institute at Memphis
Memphis, TN

Technical Institute, Oklahoma State
  University
Oklahoma, City, OK

Texas State Technical Institute
Waco, TX

Tulsa Junior College
Tulsa, OK

* Some schools refer to their courses and degrees as Biomedical Electronics Technology or Biomedical Engineering Technology.

U.S. Army Medical Equipment &
   Optical School
Denver, CO

University of Arkansas
Little Rock, AR

University of Maine
Portland, ME

University of New Mexico
Albuquerque, NM

Utah Technical College at Salt Lake
Salt Lake City, UT

Vermont Technical College
Randolph Center, VT

Western Wisconsin Technical Institute
LaCrosse, WI

Index